Healthy Family, Healthy You

The Healthy Mama's Guide to feeding your family well - simply and sanely!

Natasha Rosenstock Nadel

Copyright © 2015 Natasha Nadel

All rights reserved. No part of the contents of this work may be reproduced or retransmitted in any form without the permission of the publisher. Contact Natasha@healthyfamilyhealthyyou.com for permission, questions and resources.

This book is not intended as a substitute for the medical advice of a physician or registered dietician. The reader should regularly consult a physician in matters relating to his/her health and particularly with respect to any symptoms that may require diagnosis or medical attention.

Cover Illustration and Design by Robyn Shrater Seemann,
RS2 Studio
Copy Editing by Mary Keltner

ISBN-13: 978-0996684200 (Natasha Nadel)
ISBN-10: 0996684204

ABOUT THE AUTHOR

Natasha Rosenstock Nadel came to this story as a journalist and the information and recommendations in this book come from a decade of research, reporting, eating, and reading; in addition to having a family she tries to feed as well as possible.

After fielding many questions from friends and family about her new vegan lifestyle and the crazy concoctions coming from her kitchen, she decided to write this book. She figured it was better to tell everyone in print, rather than in person (as this has not gone well in the past), that eating animal products causes cancer and that most "kid's food" is either empty calories or just plain harmful.

In this new world of Health Coaches taking over Registered Dieticians' territory, she's not trying to be either. However, she will claim the title **"Most Creative Problem Solver,"** given to her by Dr. Neil Barnard and his staff that ran her Physician's Committee for Responsible Medicine migraine study group.

She is currently happy to be a resource to those in her community looking to create their own healthy families - and a community of support around eating well.

Visit her at www.healthyfamilyhealthyyou.com to join the conversation and find out how Natasha can speak to your community and contribute to your transformation.

Also by Natasha Rosenstock Nadel

The Healthy Family, Healthy You Cookbook: The Healthy Mama's Guide to simple, healthy versions of your family's favorite foods

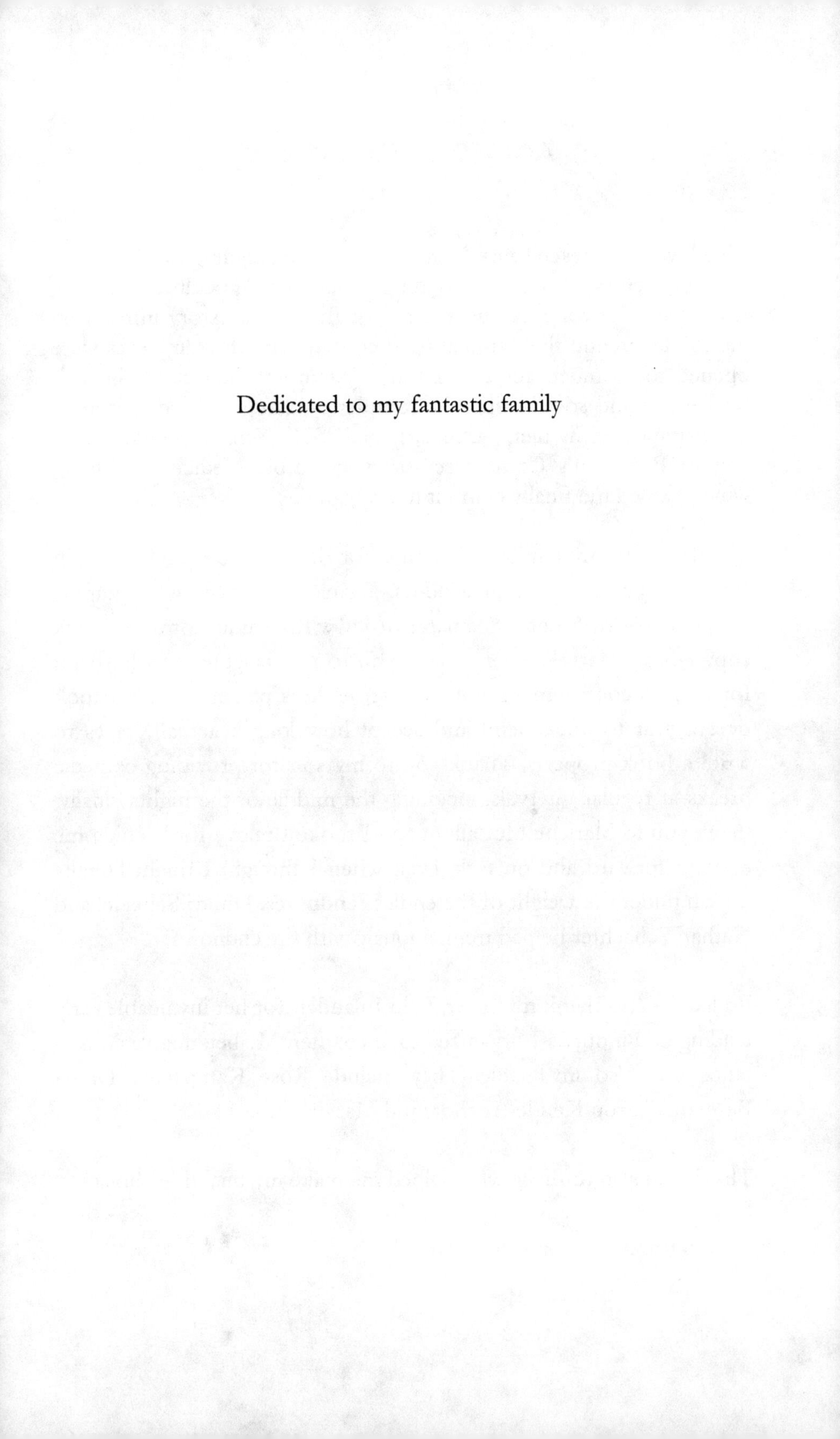

Dedicated to my fantastic family

ACKNOWLEDGMENTS

Thank you to PresenTense Magazine for first assigning me to write a magazine story about Community Supported Agriculture (CSA's), when barely anyone had ever heard of them. That story introduced me to Hazon and their annual food conference, where my eyes were opened to so much about our food system and how it fits in with Jewish law and social justice. It completely changed the direction of my writing and my diet, particularly Halè Sofia Schatz's work. Thank you to Physician's Committee for Responsible Medicine (PCRM), which helped me finally commit to a vegan diet.

Thank you to my family and friends for their support, editing, brain storming, guidance and great ideas. Thank you especially to graphic designer Robyn Shrater Seemann of www.RS2studio.com and crack copy editor, Mary Keltner. Thank you to my daughter and husband for their encouragement and (almost) endless patience while I took over a year to understand and accept how long it actually takes to write a book properly. Thank you to my son for providing comedic breaks at regular intervals, including the middle of the night. Finally, thank you to Marlene McCallum and Brooke Bralove for keeping me moving forward and on task, even when I thought I might literally drown under the weight of the endless endnotes. Dmitri Scheidel and Nathan Schachter helped tremendously with the endnotes.

I'd like to also thank my sister, Lani Inlander, for her invaluable early reading and input as I organized each chapter. My beta readers' assistance was also invaluable. They include Rose Kattezham, Dafna Berman, Sharon Kende-Anchor, and Mary Keltner.

Thank you also to those who helped me make my final title choices.

I apologize if I've forgotten anyone!

Contents

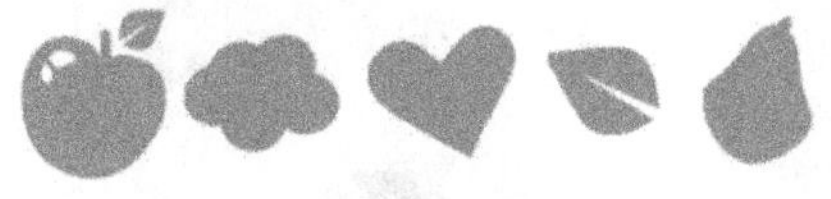

INTRODUCTION

Can't get your kids to eat healthy? Don't even know what healthy is? Worried the effort will make you crazy? In this book, I'll show you how to create a healthy family, a peaceful kitchen, and a happy you. These days, it's easy for our kids to go through an entire day without eating any fruits and vegetables. That is horrifying!

Think about it…cereal for breakfast, granola bars, crackers and cheese for snacks, pizza and potato chips for lunch, chicken nuggets and fries for dinner. Nothing green on that list, much less the 5-10 servings of fruits and vegetables they (and us, as parents) should be eating each day.

I promise you happiness and empowerment – the type of lasting happiness that comes with being clear on what you want for yourself and your family and making it happen. Get off the rollercoaster of shame and unwanted pounds - or just feeling like crap; and opt out of the constant marketing onslaught – targeted towards you and your family.

Studies show that we eat mostly the same weight in food each day. But that doesn't mean we spend our entire adult lives the same weight on the scale. I won't tell you that you need to eat "small portions," or learn to love the metallic taste of artificial sweetener in your food.

There is a different way; one in which you can eat almost as much as you want, feel satiated, improve your health and well-being and set your kids up for a healthy relationship with food; and set up your family for a long, pleasurable life together.

I know how hard it can be to change your family's eating and exercise habits. On a macro level, to transform your family's health sounds like a huge, impossible and non-specific task. That is one of the reasons why I wrote this book. I want to empower individuals and families to make doable and specific, yet substantive, changes. I also want to share why the effort is worth it and give you a road map for creating your own rewarding journey.

You care about your health and that of your family. Between busy schedules, more immediate priorities and the onslaught of processed food marketing, some days it feels like you need a full time cook if you are going to eat "real food" (that is the term I use for fruits, vegetables, legumes and whole grains, without additives). Why should you listen to me? Because that is the world I live in, too.

Perhaps everyone living in your house or in your immediate family eats the same way right now; or maybe, like in my house, you most certainly do not! Whether we are talking about your partner and kids, or your siblings and parents, I don't recommend becoming a little dictator. You can't come home one day and tell everyone that sugar is banned, and they will never see another chicken nugget again.

I'd actually be very happy if I could suddenly become the benevolent dictator of my household. Unfortunately, that probably wouldn't be very good for my marriage or my relationship with my children. So, I have taken a different tack. I replace some of the unhealthier items they like with the healthier versions, and I add whole nutrients wherever I can. In the following chapters, I will provide you with tips and tricks to do the same.

In my own family, I have had to respect that, although I'd been an on again, off again vegetarian since I was a teenager, I wasn't 'on' when I met my husband or when we got married. I was a squeamish meat eater (no bones, tongue, liver or weird animals), but I did eat it nonetheless.

About 7 years ago, after researching and writing one too many stories on the practices of the modern meat industry, I decided to re-commit to vegetarianism (pescatarianism, really, as I ate fish) once again. My conscience felt so much better. Then, while looking for healthy vegetarian recipes for my family, my friend Dafna Berman suggested I look at this new book everyone was talking about: *Eat to Live* by Dr. Joel Fuhrman.

I read about the harmful effects of all animal products, including dairy products and eggs and spent the next few years reading additional Dr. Fuhrman books and the rest of this like-minded group: Drs. Neil Barnard, T. Colin Campbell, and Caldwell B. Esselstyn, Jr, among others.

I had always said, "I believe in the food chain; I just choose not to participate in it." That's because, as a teenager, I wasn't a vegetarian because I felt sorry for the poor brown-eyed cow. I was a vegetarian because I thought animals were gross – whether cows, dogs or hamsters. As an adult, after enough research, I started caring about animal welfare and stopped believing in the typical food chain.

I gradually stopped eating eggs (unless they were cooked in something and I couldn't see them) and fish. Then I stopped eating yogurt. But cheese… ah, cheese is crack! Just like a human mother's milk that hits the pleasure centers of a baby's brain, a cow's milk hits our pleasure centers, providing dopamine to make us want more and more.

In simple terms, I could not resist pizza! Now that I don't eat it anymore, I recognize that I wanted it for that sweet spot of fatty mouth feel and salt. Somehow, that makes it easier to resist. It's like a marathon runner offered a cigarette. Why would they even want it? That is just not who they are. That's how I feel now about cheese. Like a recovering drug addict, I don't even want to go there. Umm…except when I do. I truly do see sweets and cheese as modern drugs.

New research shows that when we feel incredibly guilty about eating something we consider a treat or a cheat, it probably will make us fat. If we savor every bite and treat it with joy, it probably won't affect our waistlines. I have a new practice for myself. If I want to eat something that is a vegan treat or cheat, I am going to savor it. The thing is, most of the time it isn't worth it. So if it is worth it to me, I am going to enjoy it and not shovel it down my throat in secret. I am okay with being 90%. There are few people who can do more. If it really is a rare treat, and my head is in the right place, I don't think it will send me on a binge. I feel too good from eating well to do that.

While writing *Healthy Family, Healthy You,* I have remained conscious that I don't want to have the *Skinny Bitch* effect on my readers. As you may or may not recall, the first *Skinny Bitch* book first came out a few years ago, and the authors have written a number of offshoots since. Until readers started reading the book, they had no idea they'd be told that the only way to be skinny and moral was to stop eating animal products. Readers felt assaulted. I still liked the books because

I was personally open to the message (and recipes!). However, that first book essentially told readers that the most important priority is to avoid animal products at all costs (even though many of the faux meat products they recommend are not healthful). If you don't, you are a cruel person. In addition, the book's authors imply that part of the unhealthiness that comes along with eating animal products is the bad karma from your behavior. This was not exactly the way to win friends and admirers…

I would never tell my dear readers that they are cruel and callous. It just isn't true. We all have complicated histories, belief systems and educations around food. It just so happens that I have re-educated myself, and I'm sharing this information with you. If the only effect of your reading this book is that you learn how to incorporate more whole, plant based foods into your diet, you will still be healthier than before you picked it up. Not everyone will want to go all the way and become vegetarian or vegan. I understand that.

Like every aspect of life, what's important is to create an intention and then fulfill it in a way that makes you feel happy and whole. With consistency, you can make a big difference in your family's intake of valuable nutrients and, therefore, future health.

It is a big deal to reject the Standard American Diet (also known as SAD in plant eating circles). For instance, T. Colin Campbell, PhD, and Caldwell B. Esselstyn, Jr., M.D. (one of Bill Clinton's cardiologists, incidentally) grew up on farms. Today they are leading voices in the plant based diet movement. Do you know how much scientific evidence it must have taken for them to change the belief systems in which they were raised? The one that said meat and dairy were the foundations of a healthy diet? The one that said their families' way of life built America's health? In addition, it must have been solid evidence because they are scientists themselves. I would venture to say that most people reading this book will not require as much of a shift as they did. You won't have to wake up one day and say, "Oh my goodness, my whole life and everything I have espoused and worked for is a lie." After you watch the film *Forks over Knives*, a catalyst for many who have transformed their diets the last few years, you will understand more about these men and where they came from and how far afield they have gone.

In *Healthy Family, Healthy You* I have written vegan this and vegan that. Really, what I am talking about is a whole foods plant based [WFPB] diet. I can make vegan cinnamon buns all day, but that isn't going to contribute towards my health and longevity. So please excuse the shorthand when I simply write "vegan." I am not trying to push an agenda or dogma on my readers; only health. On the other hand, the way the modern meat and dairy industries function does bother me. It is cruel to animals and results in an increasingly unhealthy product for the consumer. I have also intentionally stopped buying makeup and beauty products that test on animals.

However, in *Healthy Family, Healthy You*, I focus on the health issues surrounding eating animal products. I am not here to tell you that your beliefs are immoral. That is counter-productive. In addition, I don't think it is morally and physically superior to eat potato chips because they're vegan. It is not about vegan in that case. It is about health. However, even with clean and humanitarian practices, I still believe that animal products are detrimental to your health (and I personally don't want anyone to kill an animal for my benefit).

In this book, you will have the opportunity to review the scientific evidence that has led me to my beliefs. Even as a long-time vegetarian, I used to think that veganism was radical and extreme, so I understand where you may be coming from as you begin to read this book. After studying this issue for a number of years, I finally made the switch. Now it feels very natural to me. It may never feel right to you, and that's ok.

In my Jewish community, many people believe a Sabbath meal is incomplete without meat and fish (unless of course you don't actually enjoy it). In this case, those foods are real delicacies and not what you eat at every meal. So savor it then, and eat your plants the rest of the week. My goal is to be at 90% with my eating goals. I think that's pretty good and much more reasonable than 100%. You need to decide what works for you. You might be surprised at what you can accomplish when you internalize the reasons for wanting to change your eating habits.

For too long, I could not commit to eliminating all animal products; a move which I had come to believe was necessary for good health. It weighed on me. Then, I had to make the commitment to someone else, not just myself. That worked. I participated in a Physicians Committee for Responsible Medicine (PCRM, Dr. Neil Barnard's organization) study on migraines. Ironically, I have to admit that eliminating all animal products did not eliminate my migraines. However, I do feel better physically. I also thought it would be a silver bullet for my stubborn post-baby weight. It wasn't, although it certainly did help and continues to help. As we would joke in our PCRM group, Twizzlers are vegan. You have to make smart choices for good health, not just avoid animal products, and darn it, I am still not perfect! Sigh… But I am on the right track and almost at my target weight, after gaining a significant amount around having my children.

After reading this book you will understand why you should SUBTRACT animal products as much as possible from your diet, and ADD whole, plant based foods. My tips, tricks and recipes will give you the tools to do this. If your belief system still tells you that you can and should eat animal products, I am not looking to change that. I am looking to improve your diet and your health.

I am not perfect and neither is my family. Just like you, I am just doing the best I can. I have found a number of ways to improve our health and I look forward to sharing those with you and your family.

I am writing this to you the same way I would speak to my own family. Right now, when they ask me questions, it goes something like this: "I think the way that I eat is healthy/ier," and I leave it at that. Sometimes they ask me additional questions, which I vaguely answer, lest I offend anyone. The questions have included, "…and you don't feel weak?" Or "But what about calcium?" and "What about iron?"

I am going to answer all of those questions, and more, in the following pages. Why is it healthier to skip animal products, and if you do, what should you be eating instead? In addition, I am going to provide you with the tools to examine your own family's health and well-being and plan for a healthy future together.

Next time you feel repeatedly pressured to eat something you don't want to eat (whether you are full or you just don't think that the food will make you feel good), try this script: "Let's make a deal: I won't encourage you to eat more than you want to, or eat food that doesn't make you feel good, if you will do the same for me. Sound good?"

At the end of the day, I hope my presentation of dispassionate scientific evidence will give you the tools with which to start an important conversation in your own home and community.

I am asking you to help me build a community of parents who support one another; and share advice, recipes and healthy meals. In high school, if you needed something, you could call your best friend and she'd be over in 10 minutes. In college, you could walk down the hall or talk to your roommate.

As a grown up with a family, we can feel isolated in our own homes. I am privileged to live in a community where my friends are in close physical proximity to one another, as our Sabbath observance requires us to walk to synagogue. However, even if you live close to one another, your best girlfriends probably have children and other responsibilities and can't just come help you at the drop of a hat.

I want to change that. Let's put one another higher up in the priority list. Transform an experience from lonely to fun by doing it together. Get your families together to cook dinner, even in the middle of the week. When you have one another over to eat, feed everyone fun, but healthy, food.

My friends are grateful that they can send their kids over to me and they know they won't be given mounds of corn syrup and artificial food coloring. In the same vein, they tell me that when they come over and I serve them delicious, filling, healthy food, a huge burden is lifted off of them. By creating a supportive environment, they don't have to make difficult decisions. They can just enjoy themselves. A whole level of stress and guilt is removed. What if we could do that for ourselves, our friends and for our larger community?

We can. After you read the book, don't forget to tell me how you have transformed your own families and communities. Let me know how else 7I can help!

Yours in health,
Natasha Rosenstock Nadel
Potomac, MD
August 2015

p.s. In this book I often refer to Mom as the primary parent preparing food and managing this aspect of the household (and the parent reading this book). I know that's not the case in every family (nor should it be!). If that is not the case in your home, please excuse my shorthand. It is only for the sake of brevity that I usually refer to Mom.

p.p.s. Grammar disclaimer. I claim to be a stickler for grammar. However…I am using healthy to describe food items that cannot be *healthy* because they are not living. The correct term is *healthful.* The reality is that in every day conversations, most people use the term healthy to describe food that should be described as health*ful.* In order to avoid sounding awkward, in this case, I am simply going with the colloquialism.

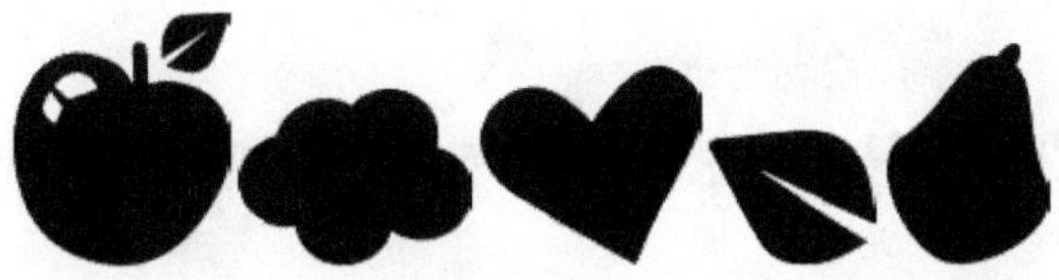

1

CASE STUDIES

Dana and Paul – Using plant power to run marathons

In her own words.

The Change

I have been a vegetarian since November 2011. My journey towards a plant based diet resulted from experimenting with dietary changes while training for my first marathon. I felt that the proteins I craved were more from vegetarian sources than meat sources. If I indulged in the vegetarian protein sources, there was no room in my belly for the meat proteins. The vegetarian tastes won out, and I eventually phased out meat altogether.

Now

I am definitely still on a journey exploring ways to incorporate even more vegan recipes into my diet and am not totally vegan -- but that was never the plan. I have phased out most dairy products and eat products that may contain eggs, but am not really eating eggs on their own anymore.

Family

A vegetarian diet definitely works for our family. My husband was only eating meat on Shabbat (Jewish Sabbath) for many years and then transitioned to being completely vegetarian. The kids have adjusted but will still eat meat when they can! Thank goodness for meat eating friends and neighbors who host them.

Friends

When we have company, guests are pleasantly surprised how well you can eat as a vegetarian.

Health

Our health and energy levels are also great. I don't know if this is clearly related to the vegetarian diet, but we definitely get a lot more vitamins and minerals from our plant based foods.

Future

The diet gives me the energy I need to train for my marathons. I have run 5 thus far. As long as I can keep running, I feel as though the fuel I am giving my body is definitely helping me achieve my fitness goals and I stay motivated to continue eating this way.

Heidi and William - Aware and at peace

In her own words.

History

My husband and I have been following a vegan diet together for four years. Before that, I was vegetarian for 20 years, and he was a total carnivore!

I first became a vegetarian for health reasons; and an awareness of our place in the food chain and not feeling comfortable with it; not thinking that just because we could kill, cook and eat an animal, we should; it just grossed me out. I still don't understand how people think that's a good idea.

It was early in college when I became vegetarian. I was finding out that there were other ways to live, and I thought it was brilliant. Growing up I never met a kid who was vegetarian, and clearly, I never met a vegan. I did not even know you could raise a child vegetarian. However, my parents were incredibly supportive.

The Change

Our plan was to raise our two girls vegetarian. Then, our younger daughter, now 11 years old, had a bunch of food allergies as a little girl. She was off dairy at 15 months, and by two and a half, she was off all animal products. So she was the original vegan in the family!

Three years ago, we were in Barnes and Noble when William handed me the Engine 2 diet book [see Resources]. He thought it would be worthwhile to adopt that kind of lifestyle and asked if I would do it with him. I thought that was thrilling. We bought it and came home. I read it that night. He was sitting next to me doing work stuff, and I was reading him the book. The author suggested that if you are a carnivore, spend a week living as a vegetarian. If that works, go to vegan. If you are already a vegetarian, you can go overnight. The next day I was vegan. That was it. Then we were both vegan and still are.

Family

Our 13 year old (the one without the food allergies) is vegetarian but not vegan. She doesn't eat fish, chicken or meat, but does eat dairy and eggs. For the most part, our house is almost entirely vegan. But if she's at a party and gets a dairy candy or something…or we are at Breadsmith buying challah without eggs and she asks for a muffin made with eggs... I don't say no. However, I don't buy eggs, cheese or dairy yogurt. Anything like that she can eat when she's out. I tell her I don't want to open the fridge door and see a carton of eggs.

She was 9 when we went vegan. She felt it was already a thing being a vegetarian – so she was not going stricter. She's never had meat, so she's very comfortable being a vegetarian but sees no need to take it further.

Health

Since we went vegan, we both have fewer sinus issues. We both used to get much more mucus and just feel drippy. We have almost none of that now. Maybe twice a year I'll get a cold. Then it will go away and I am fine. I also have fewer stomachaches. Looking back, I don't think I was tolerating the dairy well.

Generally, we are just feeling more comfortable and more in touch and at peace with our bodies. We have more awareness. There is less just putting stuff in our mouths because everyone else is, which is kind of how our society works.

I feel lighter and more at peace. We both lost weight, an added benefit. Then I discovered how to make vegan treats, so some of it came back! However, I do try to be careful that I don't eat too much sugar.

Others

I wish that more people would give veganism a try. I feel like the people I know who do it are so happy with their decision that it seems like a shame that there aren't more people trying it. It is healthier for us as individuals and the planet. The hesitation that people have towards changing their diets can be frustrating. People assume it is just kooky or they could never do it. William was such a carnivore. If he can do it, anyone can.

Home

On eating in other people's homes: When people know you are serious and not going to eat their meat, they adjust. We've been teased, but lovingly. We do get a lot of, "I am so glad you came because it forced me to be creative." It is all meant lovingly, but it is just funny.

On having company: When people are here, they know they won't be served fish or meat. If that's a problem – don't come - but no one has ever appeared unhappy.

Marlene and Andrew – Fueling fitness, quality of life and longevity

Marlene, a life coach (www.mostpowerfullife.com), and her husband Andrew have been following a plant based diet for over 2 years.
In her own words.

The Change

It started when my husband asked someone in his workout class, who was incredibly fit, how he got his results. He suggested that we watch *Forks over Knives* [See Resources], which we did immediately. It made so much sense to us.

Health

We all eat the same way, even my 4 year old. We have all noticed improvements. I no longer have an adverse reaction to nickel. (I can wear costume jewelry that contains nickel whereas before I would get a horrendous rash/irritation/scaly skin). My blood pressure is normal (used to be borderline); my rosacea has improved dramatically; I get fewer colds, and far less mucous when I do get sick. My husband's improvements include a healthier complexion with good color. In addition, my daughter's environmental allergies seem to have improved, she gets fewer colds with less mucous, and seems to recover more quickly. We are hoping that this diet will help with her severe peanut and tree nut allergies, for which we carry epi-pens, but we have no proof of this yet. She will be retested at five years old.

Motivation

We are motivated to be healthy and live a long time ~ to see our daughter grow up and to be here for her! My mom died just before her 51st birthday (I was 27) from what I believe may have been a lifestyle-exacerbated illness (uterine cancer), and her death made me very aware of the damaging effects of a poor diet. I am motivated to help my body avoid illness that I believe is diet related, or at least diet exacerbated; type II diabetes, some kinds of cancer, heart disease, etc. I am also motivated to eat without harming other beings and have found it relatively easy to do so, which has been helpful in maintaining this lifestyle.

Now

We do occasionally make exceptions, like if an egg or dairy product is an ingredient in bread or a veggie burger. However, we never make exceptions for meat, chicken, etc.

I have found that it can be very easy to get caught up in vegan junk food - just looking for substitutes for things we can "no longer eat," and this can be a high fat, high sugar, highly processed way to eat, as well. I find it helpful to really focus on the fruits and vegetables -- we are not perfect by any means -- but I know our bodies must notice the difference!

Joel - Buff athlete using plants to fuel his power

Joel (aka – that fit guy Andrew questioned at the gym), Firefighter and Founder, "Not Your Average Vegan" Facebook page. Joel has been following a plant based diet for almost three years after coming across the movie *Forks Over Knives.*

In his own words.

Change

It made complete sense to me. I transitioned overnight. I cleaned out my cabinets the next day and gave the food to my neighbor with seven kids. I went shopping and did the best that I could as we educated ourselves.

Family

My wife is a work in progress and not as extreme as me. I lost 55 pounds within four or five months, became more active and continued to educate myself. I trained for and completed an ultra marathon. I decided to continue with it, educate and inspire others, like my wife. Her family is from West Virginia and she's always said she's a meat and potatoes girl and won't put a title on her eating habits.

Then, about 8 months into it, she transitioned to a plant based diet. She wanted to get into shape for our trip to Jamaica. So I said, "Try it for 8 weeks. If you do it for that long and don't want to continue, I'll never ask you again." She did it and then never ate meat again.

Now that I look back, my approach to her was negative. I was pushing my lifestyle on her although she met me as a meat and dairy eater. I changed overnight and expected her to change too. She taught me how to speak to people, be less abrasive. I am not religious, but I sounded like a preacher saying, "You'll go to hell if you are not vegan." She taught me that you attract more bees with honey. Lesson learned. Now I lead by example. I continue to do what I am doing, and people are attracted to it. I tell them to educate themselves before they take my word for it. I tell them about the books and movies.

My (baby) daughter is vegan by association. We decided we don't want her to feel alienated from her friends, at parties, etc… so if her friends are having cheese pizza and she wants to eat it, I am not going to deny her. I don't want her to have a negative association with food. Having vegan parents, she is going to learn the basic principles through her home experience. I even have vegan children's books. I am not trying to push her, but it definitely helps for everyone at home to be on the same page.

Work

I was a backup cook at my firehouse and told them I wasn't going to cook unless it was my food. Half the people tried it. One guy did it for 60 days and lost 15 pounds. He is an ex-college basketball player and saw the most results. However, he resumed his lifestyle when he went to a cookout and had a turkey burger. That was that and he went back. Tradition kills because they think being a man includes eating meat, sitting on the couch and talking trash and not having to worry about working out. I eat dinner with them, but I eat my own dinner. Some, for no reason, develop a negative attitude towards me because I am not like them. Food is based on heavy tradition, and if you deviate, it is not positive. Again, from that I learned not to preach my lifestyle and only to lead by example. People would say, "You can't be strong." Then you see me and I am built and confident, not a hippie, and I don't eat meat.

Now

Conformity is just so boring. The more we step away from television ads and more or less conventional doctors and dietitians' recommendations, educate ourselves; think outside the box, we can make a difference. Whether or not you want to keep eating meat and decrease your global impact, eat more fruits and vegetables.

At one point I thought I was right about consuming a high protein diet. I was stuck on that. I wouldn't be where I am today had it not been for my past experiences, so I don't judge other people's beliefs.

I am not saying that my way is better. However, if you want to try it, I'll give you the resources. I don't want to push a vegetarian enthusiast away by expressing my vegan superiority.

Nancy – Cured diabetes through diet

Nancy is a nanny/housekeeper in her late 40's. Her parents, grandparents and sister all died difficult deaths from Type 2 Diabetes. Nancy experienced gestational diabetes with all four of her pregnancies. Because of her family history, she was watching carefully and found out that after her last pregnancy, her gestational diabetes had become Type 2. That was 19 years ago. For many years she watched her sugar as it bounced between a low of 108 and finally, to a high of 136. This was about two years ago. At that point her doctor also told her that her eyesight was starting to suffer and insisted she begin diabetes medication, which she did. However, it gave her terrible headaches and upset her stomach, so much so that she could not even take it regularly until she just had to stop taking it altogether.

It was about that time that I had enrolled in the Physicians Committee for Responsible Medicine (PCRM) migraine study. It had not yet begun, and I knew they were still interviewing people for a separate study on diabetic neuropathy. I'd actually never even heard of diabetic neuropathy. At the same time, I heard they were recruiting for that study, Nancy was telling me about the pain she was having in her feet and legs and how difficult it was for her to do her job with these symptoms. I came back from PCRM and asked her if it was diabetic neuropathy. She said yes. I said, "Have I got the solution for you!"

She couldn't work out being in the study for logistical reasons. However, PCRM, being the good folks that they are, held a free class for everyone who had wanted to be in the migraine/rheumatoid arthritis or diabetes studies but weren't able to participate for one reason or another.

I'd initially told them about Nancy, hoping she could be in the study. When she couldn't, they told me to bring her to this educational evening. Not only did they explain the benefits of a plant based diet, they gave everyone who attended numerous resources, including a couple of PCRM Founder and President, Dr. Neil Barnard's books, with more explanations, recipes and a diet plan.

Nancy was motivated. Her choice was to struggle with the side effects of diabetes, like neuropathy and poor eye sight; looking forward to a future of amputations like her sister; wound care like she provided as a young girl for her grandmother; or find another way. Dr. Barnard and PCRM presented that way, and she took it.
In her own words.

The Change

First, I gave up red meat. Then I gave up chicken and started to eat fish less often. For the first month, it was very difficult. It was new, and I was starving. Then I discovered nuts. I'd never really eaten them much before. Just eating nuts in moderation helped to keep me full and still does.

For a while I still had cravings for chicken and red meat, so I would sometimes have a few bites. However, after not eating it for a few months, any time I tried to even have a bite, I would get sick.

Now

I was never really one for eggs anyway. Once in a while, I'll have a couple of bites of eggs or something with eggs in there. The only dairy I really still eat is Greek yogurt a couple of times per week, so I wouldn't declare myself vegan. I also have fish once in a while. I'd say I am mostly vegetarian with very occasional dairy, fish and eggs. Very occasional.

I make sure to eat a variety of fruits, without overdoing it, by putting in a few different types into my morning green shake. Then, everyone in my family splits it.

Family

I told my family that I have to eat this particular way right now. If they want to eat the food also, great. Otherwise, they will have to make their own meals because I can't make two. For a while I offered for them to taste what I was eating. Usually, they weren't interested. Sometimes they were, and sometimes they even liked it. Then I stopped offering. Sure enough, now my granddaughter will ask, 'Nana, what are you eating? Can I have some?' My children too, will now eat more of what I make.

Health

After 9 months or so, I did not have the pain in my feet (diabetic neuropathy). I had more energy too. I went to the doctor, and she could barely believe my blood work. Neither could I. I knew I'd been feeling so much better from eating this way, but I was shocked when I received those test results. My sugars are now at 88. That is not even a diabetic level. Technically, I don't even have it anymore. I have also lost 20 pounds during this time. Before, my weight was just going up and up.

Future

I am so relieved that I found a way to change what I thought might have to be my destiny. I don't have to suffer like my relatives did.

I hope these stories show you how others, just like you, some with more resources, some with less, made changes to their diets and how they worked it out within their family and social group. There will always be reasons *NOT* to change. I hope they won't outweigh your desire to feel great every day and live a long happy life with your family, friends and community.

I can't encourage you enough to not only set an example, but to support others around you on their own health journeys, wherever they may be on their own path. As you read *Healthy Family, Healthy You*, I hope you will discover the right journey for you.

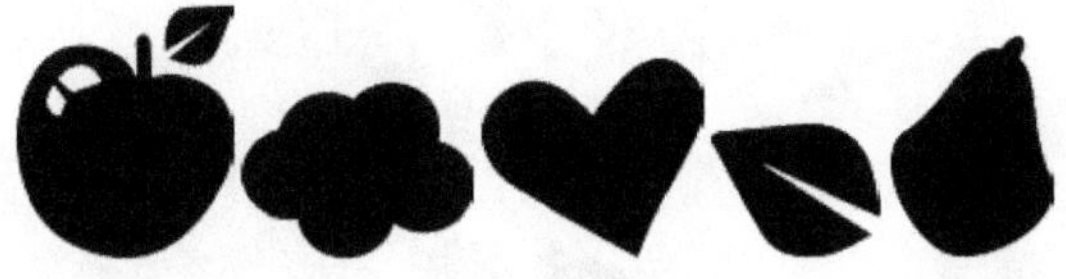

2

EVERYTHING YOU'VE LEARNED ABOUT RAISING HEALTHY KIDS IS WRONG (10 MYTHS AND FACTS)

What kind of chapter title is that? Am I trying to tell you that you are a bad mother or father? Of course not! I am trying to tell you that much of the nutritional information we take for granted as fact, is not. In fact, much of it is not even based on scientific study or evidence. It is actually based on the pressure that food industry lobbyists place on government officials.

On the positive side, many doctors, researchers, and nutritionists are promoting new, more accurate information about what is and isn't good for us. You will find information from a few of them in this chapter and you can find their books and movies in Chapter 7 (Resources).

I am about to give you a lot of information and much of it might be new for you. It might be overwhelming. You might not absorb it all the first time through. My theory here is that I can serve my audience best by giving you the relevant info in a quick and clear way. If there is a specific area in which you want more information, there are plenty of sources out there, especially those in Chapter Seven.

I have learned this information slowly, while researching every facet of nutrition, etc… over the past 10 years. I'm giving you the opportunity to just read this book and move on, without making it your life's passion or biggest hobby, like I have. As you read through the rest of the book, you may want to refer back to one or more sections, reread and review. In the meantime, I am just looking to save you time and give it to you straight. If it is a little too direct, I apologize in advance and invite you to seek out the studies and books I have cited here, for more details.

Let's review some commonly held beliefs that I'd like to challenge.

I am asserting that each one of the following "facts" is actually a "myth." I understand that you will need evidence to change your mind about information you've been given your entire life. It isn't easy to decide that the majority opinion is incorrect. Many pioneers in the research on the benefits of a whole foods plant based diet were raised on American farms. They were raised believing that their families were contributing to the health of America and Americans through their production of meat and dairy. With this background and its accompanying idealism, a young T. Colin Campbell, PhD set out to find the best way to provide protein to under-nourished children in developing countries.

Today, Dr. Campbell is the elder statesman of nutrition research, coauthor of the best-selling and influential book, *The China Study: Startling Implications for Diet, Weight Loss and Long-term Health* (BenBella Books, 2006) and wrote the New York Times Bestseller *Whole: Re-*

thinking the Science of Nutrition with Howard Jacobson, PhD. (BenBella Books, 2013).

Dr. Campbell travelled to the Philippines where the unusually high rate of liver cancer in children became part of his team's investigation. It was thought to be caused by aflotoxin, a carcinogenic mold found in peanuts and corn.

Further investigation found that the wealthier children, those with the most animal protein in their diets, were actually most likely to get liver cancer.

Surprised? Let's now review each fact/myth from the perspective of the most up-to-date scientific research. You will find more information about the animal protein and cancer link in this and the next chapter. The good news is, you will also find out how to avoid it!

~~Established Facts~~ Myths

1. Drinking milk and eating other dairy products is necessary for humans to ingest enough calcium for strong bones.

2. Using anti-bacterial soap and hand sanitizers will keep colds and flu at bay.

3. Humans (especially women and children) require red meat for adequate iron.

4. Protein is the most important nutrient for a developing child's health, and plant-based protein is inadequate.

5. The government nutritional recommendations are based on scientific evidence and safety information.

6. Poultry and fish are heart healthy.

7. Food from the children's menu is appropriate for children.

8. Bottled water is healthiest and cleanest.

9. A vegetarian diet is inherently inferior to an omnivorous one.

10. It is all about calories in, calories out.

Myth #1

Drinking milk and eating other dairy products is necessary for humans to ingest enough calcium for strong bones.

Why you believe the myth

I used to tell the standard story from one of my elementary or grade school text books. It goes like this: After Americans introduced the practice of drinking milk to Japan, post-World War II, the population grew an average of 2 inches.

I don't actually know if this is true, but it is oft-repeated. The implication is…Those ignorant Asians did not realize what they were missing. They needed to adopt the standard American diet (known as SAD in the pro-nutrition, vegan circles) of meat and milk at most meals. In listening to the more evolved and informed Americans, their nutrition improved so much that they grew taller (and taller is assumed to mean healthier, although it does not).

Fact

Americans have the highest calcium intake in the world. However, we also have one of the highest hip fracture rates in the world.[i]

Proof

According to the (somewhat famous and long-term) Nurses' Health Study, that followed 72,337 women for over 18 years, consumption of dairy does not reduce the risk of osteoporosis-related hip fractures.[ii]

Calcium, Vitamin D, and Osteoporosis

One in two women and up to one in four men over the age of 50 will break a bone due to osteoporosis.[iii] According to Dr. Joel Fuhrman, a board-certified family physician, nutritional researcher and author of four *New York Times* best-sellers about preventing and reversing disease through nutritional and natural methods, a low intake of calcium is not the primary reason so many Americans have and are at risk of getting osteoporosis. That classic American meal with a glass of milk to go with it (and the billion dollar cereal industry) has ensured that Americans have the highest calcium intake in the world. However, we also have one of the highest hip fracture rates in the world. The standard American diet encompasses too much salt, caffeine, sugar, and animal products and can cause calcium to leach out of our bones and then be lost through our urine.[iv]

Cow's milk may provide calcium, but it also provides saturated fat, hormones, antibiotics and an increased cancer risk. If you think about what you are consuming in terms of efficiency and value, there is no contest between animal and plant based calcium. Plant based sources of calcium, such as vegetables, beans, fruits, nuts, and seeds provide health-promoting minerals, fiber and antioxidants, without promoting the urinary excretion of calcium like cow's milk.[v] Vitamin K is also important for bone health and it is found in abundance in dark leafy greens.[vi]

Vitamin D

News reports abound about the benefits of Vitamin D supplementation (as we don't get enough from the sun due to environmental factors, time spent indoors, and sunscreen) for bone health, specifically in conjunction with calcium. According to Dr. Fuhrman, most Americans take inadequate amounts of Vitamin D and excessive amounts of calcium.

Biochemist Anthony Norman, an International expert on Vitamin D, reports that more than half of North American and Western Europe's population is deficient in Vitamin D.[vii] Medical studies show that Vitamin D is more effective than calcium for treating osteoporosis, as it promotes the absorption of calcium in the intestine as well as the activity of bone building cells.[viii] Ask your doctor to test your blood for Vitamin D levels and then aim for Vitamin D levels in the range of 30-45 ng/ml.[ix]

Dr. Fuhrman recommends the following:

- Limit supplemental calcium to 400-600 mg per day as studies show that 500mg prevents osteoporosis-related fractures effectively, while 1000 mg calcium does not.[x]

- Derive most of your calcium from plant foods, not supplements.

Overdosing on calcium actually deactivates the Vitamin D and can weaken bones.[xi]

Myth #2

Using anti-bacterial soap and hand sanitizers will keep colds and flu at bay.

Why you believe the myth

The ubiquitous presence of hand sanitizers in public places and products screaming "anti-bacterial"... "protect yourself and your family!"

Fact

Soap and water clean your hands better than hand sanitizer because hand sanitizer can't work if you have actual dirt on your hands. In addition, popular anti-bacterial products, including soaps, containing triclosan are ineffective against viruses (such as cold and flu) and are contributing to antibiotic resistance.

Proof

Not only does soap and water clean your hands better than hand sanitizer, recent studies show that drying your hands with a towel (sorry to all the environmentalists replacing paper towels with fancy hand dryers in public bathrooms) is an important finish to this procedure.

When you scrub your hands and rinse them under running water, the bacteria goes down the sink with the water. When you use hand sanitizer the bacteria is still on your hands. An alcohol-based hand sanitizer is better than nothing and certainly has its place and benefits. However, washing your hands for 30 solid seconds and then wiping them on a towel (paper in a public bathroom, an oft-changed cloth towel in your home) also contributes to removing any leftover dirt and bacteria.

Every time I walk by a certain shop in the mall, I lament all the customers in there, buying anti-bacterial soap and hand sanitizers that contain triclosan.

Triclosan does not protect against fungi or viruses and can also contribute to bacterial resistance, as bacteria evolves to counteract the anti-bacterial products that are now everywhere in our home, personal products and even clothing.

The medical establishment has tried to raise awareness about antibiotic resistance over the past few years. There are an increasing number of infections that doctors no longer have any tools (antibiotics) to treat.

What is your main concern about getting sick in the winter? Flu and colds, right? Those are viruses. If your sweet smelling triclosan-containing soap isn't killing the cold and flu, why would you use it and contribute to antibiotic resistance?

Oh, and before I forget, there is another reason not to use those sweet smelling soaps and sanitizers. Artificial scents present in our bath products, air fresheners, and hand sanitizers, along with triclosan, are hormone disruptors. They are suspected of contributing to obesity, early puberty, and an increase in breast cancer, among other harmful effects. [See the Resources chapter for the most important book you can read about personal care product safety (or lack thereof). That book has already been written, and very well, so I am going to try to keep to my own topic in this book!]

You can also find natural air fresheners (for the bathroom, car, kitchen, etc…) at health food stores and online. There is no reason to promote early puberty while freshening your home or taking a bubble bath with artificially scented products.

The Food and Drug Administration (FDA) is currently reviewing the potential toxicity of triclosan-containing products. In Europe and the United States, hospitals won't even use them because they don't reduce infections or illness.

Alcohol-based sanitizers that are 60% alcohol are good at killing bacterial pathogens and can also kill some viruses. One notable exception: The norovirus, responsible for the recent high-profile and disastrous cruise ship outbreaks of illness.

Just remember that the alcohol cannot magically work if there is actual visible dirt on your hands. It will simply stay on top of the dirt.

You are best off putting a strict routine into your own and your kids' heads. Wash, for 30 seconds, all over your entire hands and under nails (especially with kids!), before food preparation and after using the bathroom. Regular soap and water, naturally scented with essential oils if desired, and a hand or paper towel are our best weapons against missing work or school for illness.

Myth #3

Humans (especially women and children) require red meat for adequate iron.

Why you believe the myth

Because your grandmother grew up on this edict and is pressuring you! Seriously! As a teenager, my grandmother used to make me eat a hamburger at least 1 time a year to make herself feel better that I wasn't going to drop dead from being a vegetarian. According to a recent study, the reason for this lays in a fear that iron-deficiency anemia may lead to neuro-developmental deficiencies.

Fact

With abundant options for plant based iron-rich foods, there is no need to take on the risks of eating red meat, simply out of concern for potential infant iron deficiency.

In fact, iron from animal sources can be toxic if you ingest too much. Plant iron is eliminated once you have used what you need.

Proof

New research explains the positive role of iron-containing protein in plants while studies show that red meat consumption is linked to a sharp increase in both disease and overall mortality.[xii]

Per 100 calories, collard greens, lentils and broccoli contain significantly more iron than a hamburger. Plant based iron can be harder for the body to absorb, than animal-based iron. However, combining the plant based foods with those high in vitamin c, such as fruit, can increase absorption.

Now, let it be said here that 100 calories of hamburger is a lot less food than 100 calories of broccoli. But that is the beauty of the way I am encouraging you to eat! You can eat a lot! You can eat until you are satisfied and then still feel good about yourself physically and mentally. Imagine that!

Myth #4

Protein is the most important nutrient for a developing child's health, and plant based protein is inadequate.

Why you believe the myth

People from developing nations, many without access to animal protein, are often smaller and less healthy than their western counterparts who do consume animal-based protein.

Fact

In these developing areas, there is also poorer public health, greater childhood disease and a lack of an available variety of foods, all of which can stunt growth.

When you combine good public health, a variety of nutrients, and a good deal of plant proteins, you find that it is possible to grow just as big and tall (although, usually not as overweight) on a plant based diet.[xiii]

Proof

The China Study

The most comprehensive study of diet, lifestyle and disease ever done with humans in the history of biomedical research. It was a massive undertaking jointly arranged through Cornell University, Oxford University and the Chinese Academy of Preventive Medicine. The New York Times *called it the "Grand Prix of Epidemiology." This project surveyed a vast range of diseases and diet and lifestyle factors in rural China and, more recently, in Taiwan…this project eventually produced more than 8,000 statistically significant associations between various dietary factors and disease!*[xiv]
– T. Colin Campbell, The China Study

In the China Study, consuming more protein, of any kind, was associated with greater height and weight for men and women. T. Colin Campbell writes in his book of the same name, "However, this effect was primarily attributed to plant protein because it makes up 90% of the total Chinese protein intake."[xv]

Animal protein not only doesn't CONTRIBUTE to health, it DIMINISHES health. Too much animal-sourced protein actually promotes cancer in humans and animals. Plant based protein sources provide healthful minerals, vitamins and phytochemicals (a naturally occurring plant substance that has been shown to protect against disease).

A healthful vegetarian diet will provide plenty of protein and other vitamins and minerals. The key here is the healthful part. You can be a vegetarian who eats nothing but white bread and sugar and then you will be missing many vital minerals, including protein. If you simply drop meat products from your diet, but don't increase the amount and number of healthful foods you consume, yes, you may also be deficient in important nutrients.

In addition, nutritionists no longer believe that vegetarians must combine specific proteins to create a "complete protein." As long as you eat a varied diet, full of nutritional foods, everything you eat throughout the day should work together on its own, without being eaten in the same meal.

Now that we've established why you should NOT be concerned about getting enough protein on a vegan diet, let's talk about why you SHOULD be concerned about getting your protein from animal products.

As previously mentioned, in the 1960's Dr. Campbell went to the Philippines to work with malnourished children. This was the start of his career and he was full of idealism and eager to spread the healthy American diet to the rest of the world. However, his investigation into the high levels of liver cancer in Filipino children led him to a startling discovery.

Too much protein, specifically too much animal-sourced protein, actually *caused* cancer in his studies' subjects (human and animal).

At first, Dr. Campbell could not believe the results of his own research. This was before the China Study and his many others, at the start of his career, and contrary to everything he and his fellow scientists had been taught. According to his results, what he thought was the medicine for malnourishment (animal protein), was a poison.

After he made this surprising discovery, he found a research report from India that had found the same thing, and more. The Indian researchers administered the carcinogenic aflotoxin to two groups of rats. They then fed one group a diet of 20% protein. This is a level that matches what most Westerners eat. In the second group of rats, they fed them only 5% protein.

As Dr. Campbell writes in *The China Study*, "Incredibly, every single animal that consumed the 20% protein diet had evidence of liver cancer, and every single animal that consumed a 5% protein diet avoided liver cancer. It was a 100 to 0 score, leaving no doubt that nutrition trumped chemical carcinogens, even very potent carcinogens, in controlling cancer."[xvi]

Eventually his research into the protein-cancer link was funded for 27 years, mostly by the National Institutes of Health (NIH), the American Cancer Society and the American Institute for Cancer Research.

After all these studies and so many peer-reviewed journal articles, I agree with Dr. Campbell when he writes that despite all findings being consistent, "people are still confused." That *is* a tragedy and something he wanted to change with his 2006 book, *The China Study*. He may be doing just that, as *The China Study* appears to grow in popularity and public consciousness each year.

Here are the other relevant findings about protein from his, and many others' studies:

- Regardless of how much aflotoxin was administered to the animals, low-protein diets inhibited the initiation of cancer by this carcinogen.

- Even after the cancer had formed, low protein diets actually "dramatically blocked subsequent cancer growth."

- The cancer-producing effects of aflotixin were rendered insignificant by a low-protein diet. The researchers said they could turn the cancer on and off simply by changing the level of protein consumed.

- Not ALL proteins had this effect. **Casein, found in cow's milk protein, promoted all stages of the cancer process. Protein from plants, including wheat and soy, did not promote cancer, even at the highest levels.**

For our purposes (clarity and simplicity), and Dr. Campbell's, here is the most important summary of the China Study findings: "People who ate the most animal-based foods got the most chronic disease. Even relatively small intakes of animal-based foods were associated with adverse effects. People who ate the most plant based foods were the healthiest and tended to avoid chronic disease."[xvii]

Still think that animal-based protein is the most important nutrient for your children's growth? No one is saying children shouldn't eat protein. However, they should get it from sources that also provide them with actual nutrients that will make them healthier. Animal protein not only doesn't CONTRIBUTE to health, it DIMINISHES health. Now, why wouldn't our government tell us that? That brings us to our next myth.

Myth #5

The government nutritional recommendations are based on scientific evidence and safety information.

Why you believe the myth

We are Americans and we like to think that our government is always looking out for our well-being, over that of corporations.

Fact

Many scientists involved in government recommendations on diet have a clear conflict of interest as they either have worked for food industry groups or currently consult for them.

Proof

In the 1980's, one day you might have seen a report released from a government committee that linked a high-fat diet to cancer; while the next day, you might see a scientist on the news extolling the health of McDonald's hamburgers. In fact, that scientist on the news could be both on the government payroll, and that of many major food industries, such as eggs and dairy. The conflicts of interest are clear, as is the confusion caused to the public.

Here are two examples[xviii]:

In one case, a Public Nutrition Information Committee report alleged that low-fat diets are fraudulent scams, while the National Academy of Sciences reported the opposite.

In another, the American Cancer Society gave almost no credence to the idea that diet is linked to cancer, while the American Institute for Cancer Research reported that it is indeed linked.

My plate vs. pcrm power plate

A few years ago, PCRM sent the federal government their idea for replacing the traditional food pyramid.

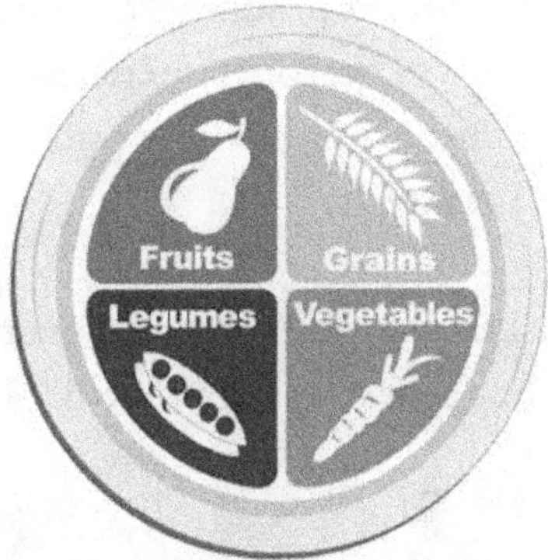

You probably know what the government ultimately released in 2011.

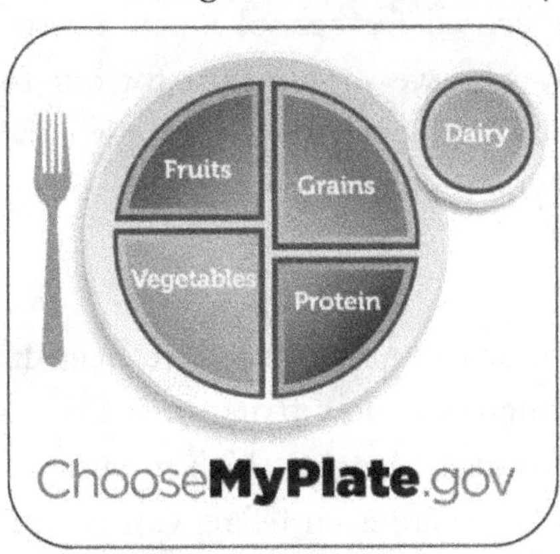

The USDA replaced LEGUMES with PROTEIN and added a circle reminiscent of a drinking glass and/or yogurt cup for DAIRY. Can you imagine the lobbying that must have gone into that plate? Dairy, Beef, Poultry and probably even Processed Foods lobbies must have been banging down the door on the USDA. I actually feel sorry for the government officials under so much pressure and scrutiny! But, that doesn't mean I agree with what they chose. Why choose "protein" without fiber and micronutrients (such as animal-based protein sources), when you can eat legumes, which are disease-fighting super stars?

Processed food products

Isn't it an American freedom to choose to kill oneself with donuts? Of course it is. The problem is we are not really talking about "food" here. We're talking about food products, food coloring, food preservatives, etc… There is no reason Americans should have to eat chemicals banned in other parts of the world. Can you imagine the following scenario in France?

In 2007, Frito-Lay asked the FDA for permission to label Fritos as "heart healthy" and the request was approved![xix] Enough said?

School lunches

When the United States Congress counts pizza as a vegetable and allows fries to be served for school lunch, every single day of the week, is this really who we should trust for our food recommendations? Do you think our politicians are simply concerned with children's health or do you think they might be receiving just a *teensy* bit of industry pressure?

Although school lunch requirements have been improved over the past few years, Congress is now trying to gut that legislation and go back to entirely processed lunches, high in fat and sodium. Some of the big food companies are even telling Congress that they want the improvements rolled back because the "lunch ladies'" morale takes a beating every time a child throws out the fresh fruits and vegetables from their lunch trays. Just because your child doesn't want healthy food the first couple of times you give it to them, doesn't mean you start giving them pizza and fries for every single meal. Yet that is what food companies are telling Congress to do.

Let's Move

Notice that Michelle Obama's (laudable) fight against the epidemic of childhood obesity puts the responsibility for this situation squarely at the feet of the children who see over 1000 advertisements for fast food per year[xx] (this doesn't even count the advertisements they see for regular old junk food found in the grocery store rather than a fast food restaurant). It is because of government policies and subsidies that these same children are eating pizza and fries for lunch every day and suffering the consequence of the daily reality for parents on a tight budget: healthy and fresh = expensive and processed and fattening = cheap.

Instead of taking food companies to task, Let's Move implies that the rise in obesity in children is mostly due to a lack of exercise. While making changes to our sedentary society is absolutely part of the solution, I hardly think it is the biggest reason for the obesity crisis in this country. By focusing on exercise, Mrs. Obama is able to bypass much food industry pressure.

Myth #6

Poultry and fish are heart healthy.

Why you believe the myth

The popularity of "The Mediterranean Diet" and the barrage of advertising promoting poultry as a healthy alternative to red meat.

Fact

Chicken is not a harmless substitute for red meat. No one "needs" to eat poultry to be healthy. It is not essential for children or adults. In fact, its numerous toxicities make it harmful. Both 4 ounces of beef and 4 ounces of chicken contain approximately 85 milligrams of cholesterol.[xxi] In addition, while fish does contain omega-3 fatty acids essential to human health, its high levels of environmental toxins make it too polluted to rely on for this purpose. A clean algae-based supplement and nuts and seeds are better choices.

Proof

Most people know that red meat contains cholesterol and is not heart healthy. However, the common myth that chicken is heart healthy is incorrect, as is the myth that eating a turkey burger is a healthy alternative to a beef burger. Most turkey burgers are made with dark meat, comparable in fat and cholesterol levels to most beef. It may contain less saturated fat than dark meat or beef, but even the white meat in chicken and turkey contains cholesterol. A 3 oz serving of white meat turkey (and we know that most real-life servings are at least twice that) provides 16-25% of the government's upper limit of allowable cholesterol, 300 mg. (As an aside, any cholesterol in our diets is harmful and unnecessary. The 300 mg number the government came up with is meaningless, or perhaps the result of food industry pressure).

According to the National Chicken Council, Americans eat the most chicken of any country in the world at 84 pounds of chicken per person a year.[xxii] That large number is the reason that 8 *billion* chickens are slaughtered in the United States each year.[xxiii] Each year the U.S. Department of Agriculture is inspecting fewer and fewer of those chickens, while your risk of getting sick increases.[xxiv]

Here are a few reasons NOT to eat chicken:

- Chickens can soak in "fecal soup" for up to an hour before being packaged for consumers.[xxv]

- Peracetic acid and chlorine are both commonly used to treat chicken for contaminants in poultry plants.[xxvi]

- Nearly 75 percent of bacterially tainted chicken products harbor germs resistant to one or more types of antibiotics (super-bugs).[xxvii]

- Arsenic (a carcinogenic put into chicken feed to kill bacteria, make them grow bigger and the meat more pink) in chicken could lead to increased risk of lung and bladder cancer deaths.[xxviii]

Myth #7

Food from the children's menu is appropriate for children.

Why you believe the myth

Because every school lunchroom and children's menu offers the same thing: hot dogs, fries, pizza, and chicken nuggets. These have become ingrained in our brains as "children's food." They get used to it and that is all they want.

Fact

These options are fattening, fried, gross, and contribute to cancer, obesity and Type 2 diabetes.

Proof

The usual choices of macaroni and cheese, chicken nuggets, a hot dog and fries, makes the other usual children's menu choices of pea-nut butter and jelly (with high fructose corn syrup) on white bread and white spaghetti and tomato sauce (again, probably with high fructose corn syrup and a ton of sodium) sound as good as a green smoothie!

The above options have several qualities that are horrible for your children (and you, too, when you finish off their plate!).

We've already discussed the cancer causing properties of milk and other animal protein above.

Let's turn to the harmful effects of fat (I'm looking at you, macaroni and cheese, bologna, hot dogs, hamburgers and other kids' meal favorites).

With a few healthy exceptions (such as avocados, nuts and seeds), animal-based foods are much higher in fat than plant based foods. In fact, if you compare the amount of fat in the diets of different countries, it is almost a perfect correlation to the amount of animal-based foods they consume.[xxix]

Dietary fats contribute substantially to the risk of several forms of cancer (breast, colon, prostate, and others), heart disease, diabetes, gallstones, and numerous other problems as well. Although animal fats are the worst, vegetable oils also increase health problems (The good fats found in whole foods, such as avocados, nuts and seeds are an exception.).[xxx]

Let's move on to the dangers of fried foods, such as chips and fries. Foods (both processed and at home) that are baked (enough to produce browning) or fried at high temperatures can produce high levels of cancer-causing chemical compounds called acrylamides.

Unfortunately, acrylamides also form in other foods, such as breakfast cereals, and any foods you bake until brown or fry at home.

However, if you steam or boil those foods, the compounds will not form.[xxxi]

And finally, the gross:

Chicken Nuggets: Head, Shoulders, Knees, and Toes

"Researchers in Mississippi dissected chicken nuggets from two national fast-food chains and determined that chicken nuggets are a mixture of blood vessels, nerves, muscle, cartilage, fat, and pieces of bone."[xxxii] Ask your children if that sounds appetizing to them!

Myth #8

Bottled water is healthiest and cleanest.

Why you believe the myth

Relentless advertising from multi-national corporations.

Fact

We have no reason to think (besides advertising) that bottled water is safer than your average tap water. The government has practically no oversight (one person at the FDA, who has bottled water in her portfolio, among other responsibilities) on the bottled water industry. There is no testing required, whereas municipal water needs to be tested multiple times a day for contaminants.

Proof

There are so many problems with bottled water, from start to finish, that once you have learned more about them, you will be running to buy reusable metal or glass water bottles to fill with filtered water (from your own faucet!) for your family.

One leading issue: Bisphenol A (BPA) is a chemical found in most hard plastics, including plastic water bottles and 5 gallon water jugs.

Until recently (because of public outcry) it was also found in baby bottles and baby formula packaging.

According to the Environmental Working Group, "BPA is a synthetic estrogen that can disrupt the endocrine system, even in small amounts. It has been linked to a wide variety of ills, including infertility, breast and reproductive system cancer, obesity, diabetes, early puberty, behavioral changes in children and resistance to chemotherapy treatments."[xxxiii]

Most water bottles are now made from PET, a petrochemical plastic. BPA has been removed from many water bottles, but it is still present in 5 gallon jugs in most offices.

The problems with bottled water begin with its extraction. Much of the bottled water in the United States is actually just filtered municipal water. You know…like the kind you can get from your own tap! Other "spring" water is taken from different areas around the United States and then trucked to distribution sites. Besides the environmental impact of the gasoline used to ship a commodity that most Americans already have in their own kitchens (which they can further filter if needed or desired), there is also an impact on the local communities.

According to the documentary "Tapped," (2009) 40% of bottled water is drawn from municipal sources. What many companies do (the big three are Nestle, Coke and Pepsi) is buy a piece of land and tap the water table from there in unlimited amounts. In "Tapped" a community is shown in the throes of a drought that is wreaking havoc on the local economy. However, the corporation just keeps sucking up water from the little piece of land they bought under the radar and trucking it away. There is no law against tapping a well on your own property. It costs them 6 cents a gallon to extract and they sell it for 6 dollars a gallon.

Only 20% of bottles are recycled. The rest end up in landfills and the ocean. Due to the bottling plant there, the people of Corpus Christi, Texas must live with benzene (a carcinogenic, colorless, flammable, toxic liquid with a distinct odor) emissions and toxic fumes, higher rates of cancer and other illnesses. They can't even sell their homes to get away from the pollution because no one wants to buy a home next to the plant.

Bottled water is an over 10 billion dollar industry. While a few of us trying our best to minimize our bottled water consumption may not eliminate the demand for it, we can at least know we are not contributing to the environmental damage it causes and that we are ingesting fewer chemicals.

Myth #9

A vegetarian diet is inherently inferior to an omnivorous one.

Why you believe the myth

The continued proliferation of outdated scientific research.

Fact

Vegetarian foods DO NOT need to be combined in a specific way to create a "complete protein." In addition, much of the supplementation suggested for vegetarians applies to most Americans.

Proof

While it is true that people who don't consume animal products need to take a B12 supplement, it is also true that so does everyone over 50, at which time we can no longer digest the B12 from animals anymore.

In addition, this is not proof that the world was designed for everyone to eat meat. B12 used to be present in the soil, before much of it degraded due to environmental factors. Finally, people used to eat more dirt with their vegetables. These days, most food that comes from the ground is washed thoroughly before we ever see it in the super market. Then we wash it again. (I am NOT suggesting you change this routine!).

B12 is available as a supplement and also from fortified plant milks, nutritional yeast, and fortified cereals. All B12 vitamins sold meet the minimum requirement of 2.4 micrograms per day (so feel free to buy the cheapest one!). In addition, it is water soluble, meaning that we eliminate what we don't need, so there aren't any worries about over-dosing.

Until very recently, nutrition experts thought that vegetarians had to *combine* certain types of food within one meal in order to *create* a *complete* protein, to *compensate* for their diet deficient in animal products. This is no longer the case. As long as vegetarians/vegans eat a range of foods throughout the day, they will be quite complete and healthy. Beans, grains, vegetables and fruit all contain protein and provide as much as needed. (Incidentally, quinoa, the South American seed growing exponentially in popularity, is considered a complete protein.)

Myth #10

It is all about calories in, calories out.

Why you believe the myth

Previous scientific consensus.

Fact

Your body processes real food calories much more efficiently than processed and fake food calories. That is why people who drink diet soda often GAIN weight. In addition, when you have eaten real food your body understands you have eaten and you feel full, suppressing the desire to over-eat and cravings for junk food. When you eat fake food, your cravings increase. When you eat "diet" fake food (the worst type of processed food), you are left both unsatisfied *and* wanting more, with a body that doesn't know what to do with the artificial food's calories. So they sit in your butt, your stomach and your thighs.

Proof

The China Study compared data from Chinese office workers (the least active people in China) with average Americans. "Average calorie intake (per kilogram of body weight) was 30% *higher* among the least active Chinese than among average Americans. Yet body weight was 20% *lower*."[xxxiv] The Chinese low-fat, low-protein diet of whole foods shifts conversion of calories from storage as fat, to burning off as body heat and to run other body functions and systems.[xxxv]

Counting Calories and Carbohydrates

Over the last 15 years I have observed two particular schools of thought regarding calories. The first is that one must count every calorie and stay below a certain level (say, 1500 calories) to lose weight. This brings with it measuring portions of everything from coffee creamer to lettuce. Approximately eight years ago, in an attempt to truly know the number of calories I was consuming (and to control that number; of course), I bought a digital food scale that tells me how many calories are in hundreds of foods. I would place an apple on it and be disappointed that it was actually 200 calories and not the 100 estimated, without regard to size, in calorie count books. A person can make themselves nuts, limiting foods to specific portions, all day. For me, the worst part was that I was always hungry! I found it impossible to subsist on 1400-1500 calories per day, by eating super small portions of the usual foods.

The second school of thought is that, as long as you avoid carbohydrates (like the Atkins Diet), you can eat however much you want. Have that 12 oz steak. Just don't eat the baked potato on the side.

Yes, people can lose weight this way, but they often feel like crap (specifically, fatigued and constipated), go off the wagon and gain it all back. It is also important to remember that losing weight at all costs is not the object of this exercise. It is to be *healthy*. I remember a friend on Atkins once telling me that she could not eat any fruits and vegetables for the first week or two because they contained carbohydrates. That did not make sense to me from any stand point of health. You can also lose weight eating only 5 low fat, fake food chocolate pudding cups every day. It doesn't mean you should or that it will be good for your health.

Unfortunately, this cycle is the result for many of us when we eat in the typical western way:

Eating Low Nutrient Foods
SAD
(Standard American Diet)
Poor Health and Weight Gain
Overeating and Food Cravings

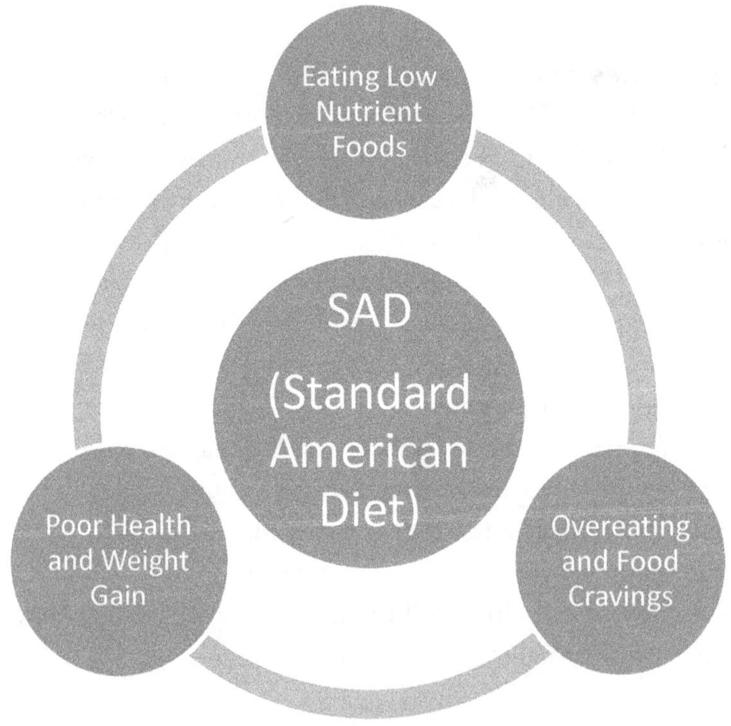

Dr. Neil Barnard is a nutrition researcher, author, health advocate and president and founder of Physician's Committee for Responsible Medicine (PCRM). Growing up in Fargo, N.D., his extended family includes both doctors and cattle ranchers, two groups that are increasingly butting heads over America's health policies. Dr. Barnard's scientific approach aims to shed new light on these important issues.

Dr. Barnard's book, "Foods that cause you to lose weight: The Negative Calorie Effect" asserts that high protein diets are dangerous and that carbohydrates actually help you *lose* weight.[xxxvi] This was first published in 1992 and has been reprinted several times since. However, the information still isn't out there in a big enough way.

I am going to do my best to break it down for you here.

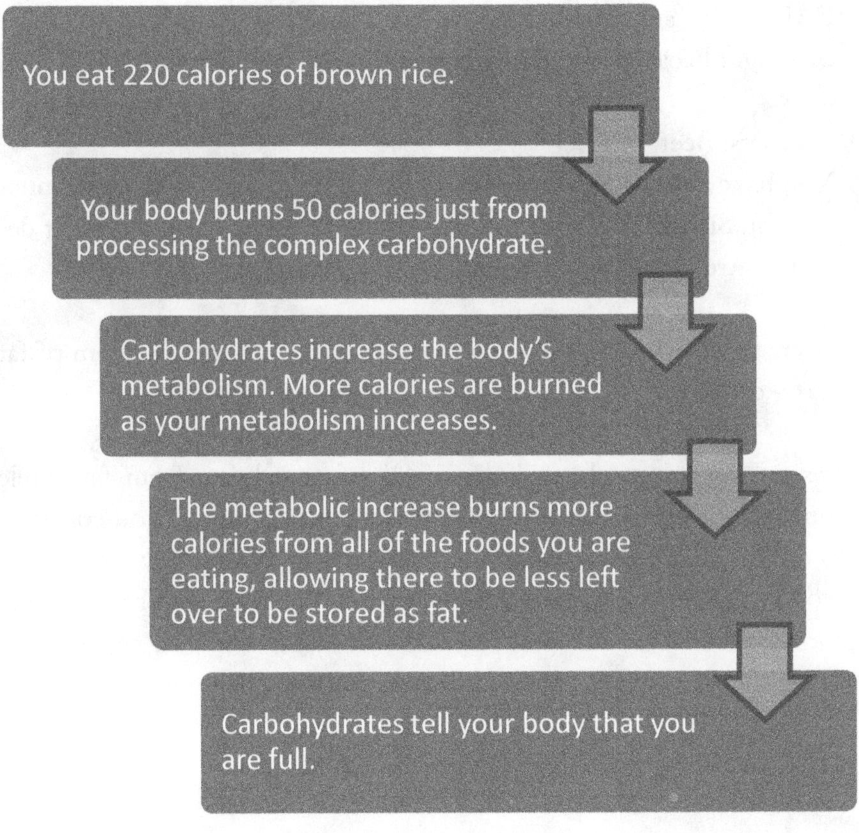

You eat 220 calories of brown rice.

Your body burns 50 calories just from processing the complex carbohydrate.

Carbohydrates increase the body's metabolism. More calories are burned as your metabolism increases.

The metabolic increase burns more calories from all of the foods you are eating, allowing there to be less left over to be stored as fat.

Carbohydrates tell your body that you are full.

(By the way, keeping food as close to its original form, like eating wheat berries vs. white flour, increases the number of calories your body burns to process the food).

Fat

People always ask me, "Well, what about extra lean ground beef or a boneless breast of chicken? What's wrong with that?"

Advertisers always have a trick up their sleeves. Here are a few great examples that Barnard uses to illustrate the confusion over fat.

Fat is often described by percentage of weight, not calories.

2% milk is 2% fat by WEIGHT. In reality, 35% of the milk's CALORIES are from fat. Does that sound low fat to you? It is 2% by weight because of the weight of the water in the milk!

Beans vs. Beef

You have a decision to make. You are going to make tacos for dinner tonight. Should you use extra lean ground beef or black beans? It depends. Are you trying to lose weight or gain it?

A gram of carbohydrate (such as beans) has 4 calories. A gram of fat has 9 calories.

Extra lean ground beef derives 54% of its calories from fat, while only 4% of beans' calories are from fat. In one meal, if you consume 3 ounces of the taco filling (and really, who is eating only 3 ounces?), you can choose between 225 calories for the extra lean ground beef or 80 calories for the beans. Besides the calories coming in, consider what they're doing once they get there (inside your body).

Carbohydrates result in the production of two natural hormones, norepinephrine and thyroid hormone (T3), both of which increase your metabolism.

Carbohydrates are only found in plants.

Animal fat is a calorie storage area for animals. Is that something you need in your body? What does that do for you? I'll tell you: It puts fat ON YOU, and promotes obesity, cancer, heart disease and diabetes.

In addition, a new meta-analysis published by the Canadian Medical Association, found that LDL ("bad") cholesterol dropped an average of 5 percent after consuming half a cup of beans per day for an average of six weeks.[xxxvii] Now, do you choose the "extra-lean" ground beef or the beans?

Meat encourages your body to store fat. Although nuts and seeds are denser in calories, studies show that they promote weight loss and general health.[xxxviii]

Your body does not actually absorb all of the fat and calories in seeds and nuts. In addition, unhealthy fats bind to the seeds and nuts, pulling cholesterol out of your body through elimination. The good fats stay in your body to provide positive health benefits.[xxxix]

The way of eating that I am suggesting *does* cut out certain food groups as Atkins does. However, it cuts out the food groups that don't actually provide you with the phytochemicals and nutrients that promote health and longevity. In addition, you can eat as much as you want of the following four food groups (and you will feel energetic, instead of miserable!): fruits, vegetables, whole grains and legumes. And you won't be miserable. That is because real food, especially food with fiber, like the aforementioned four groups, helps regulate blood sugar and cravings. You won't want to over-eat real food, once the toxic fake food is out of your system.

In the book, "Salt, Sugar, Fat: How the Food Giants Hooked Us" by Michael Moss, the author explains how the processed food you like, often sold to you as healthy, is engineered in a LABORATORY to hit the bliss centers of your brain (like illegal drugs) and to bypass the natural censors in your brain and stomach that tell you when you are full.[xl]

After reading that book, I felt like such a sucker. There are so many people that feel badly about themselves. With slogans, and scientific study, designed to make sure "you can't eat just one," we shouldn't be making ourselves feel badly over our lack of self-control. We should be avoiding the foods that upset our bodies' and our brains' natural balance, often causing cravings while taking away satiation.

I have several recommendations for you that are not simply about removing animal products from your diet to become vegetarians or vegans. Twizzlers are vegan. That doesn't mean they're good for you. While I believe, and evidence shows, that all animal products are detrimental to your health, that doesn't mean that all non-animal products are good for you. That is where making smart choices and eating real food comes in.

The Old Way

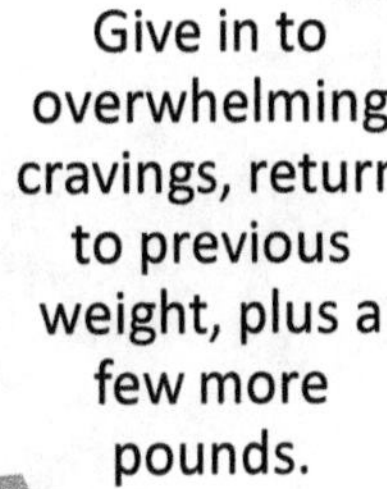
Give in to overwhelming cravings, return to previous weight, plus a few more pounds.
The Failed Diet Cycle
Turn low self-esteem into determination to restrict your food and lose weight
Limit portion sizes and count calories

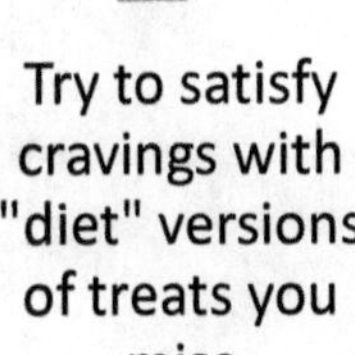
Try to satisfy cravings with "diet" versions of treats you miss

This is the world I try to stay within and one I hope you will give a try too, especially after taking advantage of the resources in this book.

The New Way

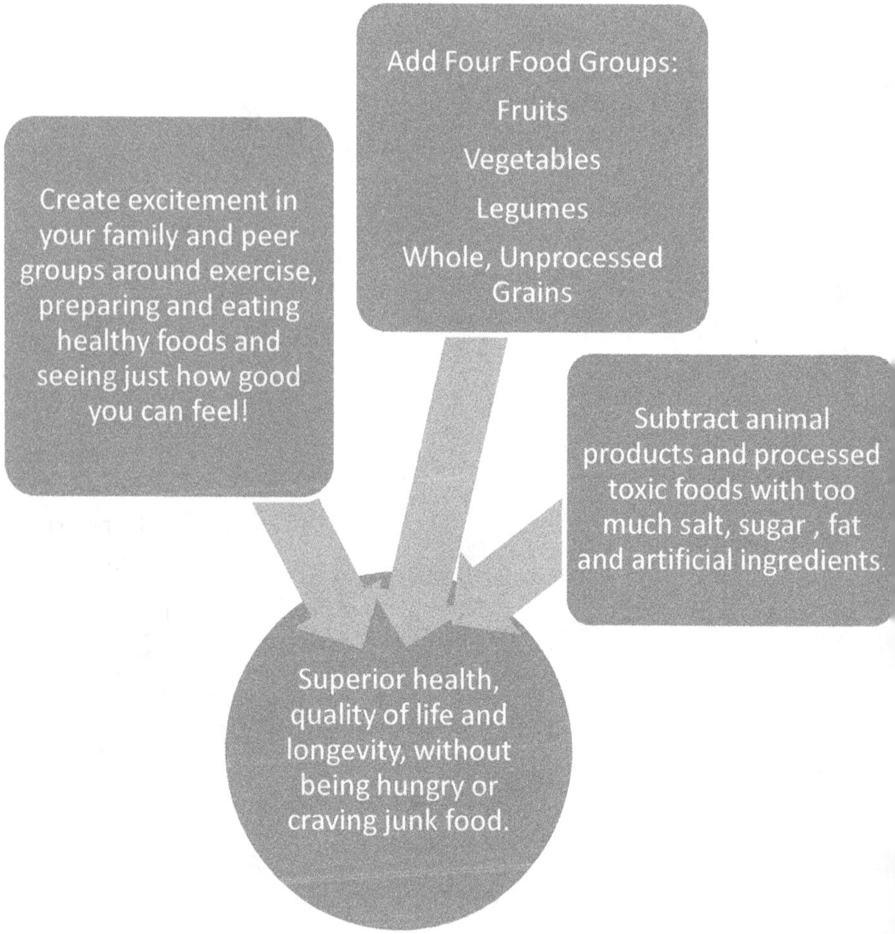

Add Four Food Groups:
Fruits
Vegetables
Legumes
Whole, Unprocessed Grains

Create excitement in your family and peer groups around exercise, preparing and eating healthy foods and seeing just how good you can feel!

Subtract animal products and processed toxic foods with too much salt, sugar , fat and artificial ingredients.

Superior health, quality of life and longevity, without being hungry or craving junk food.

You can do it!

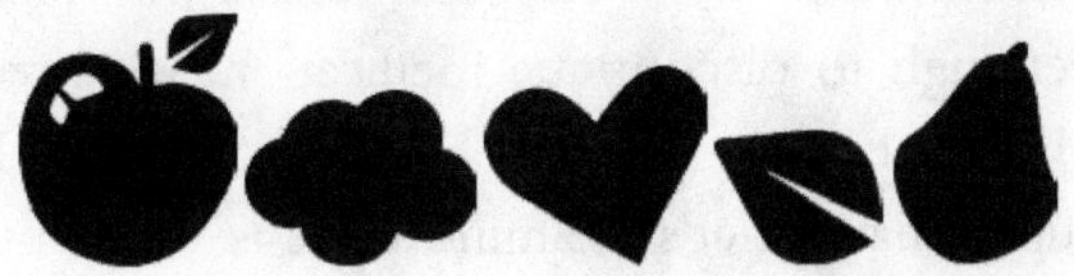

3

THE EFFECTS OF LIFESTYLE AND DIET ON HEALTH AND DISEASE

You have great power to change your health by eating well. Many doctors say their patients don't see great results with dietary changes, at least not enough to discontinue medication. However, pro-plant doctors like Joel Fuhrman, Caldwell Esselstyn, Jr., Neil Barnard, and John McDougall, have. Let's examine what is different about their approach.

If your doctor told you that you could solve your diabetes, high blood pressure or heart disease, on your own, through dietary changes, wouldn't you want to go for it? If your doctor told you that they had hundreds or thousands of patients who had avoided surgery and a life only half-lived due to ill health, through these specific dietary changes, wouldn't you become excited, want to know everything, and try to make drastic changes so that you too could receive these results?

Unfortunately, doctors are trained to solve health problems primarily through prescription drugs and surgery. Few receive any meaningful nutrition education. Few have witnessed the dramatic improvements possible through a change in diet. If you or someone you love is suffering from chronic disease, you have a right to know what works.

Many doctors don't encourage patients to change their lifestyle as drastically as needed because they simply don't have faith that they will actually do it. In their view, if you have already seriously progressed into the disease, the dietary change necessary to improve to the point of STOPPING MEDICATION, is just too much for the average American.

But what if you *aren't* the average American and you are willing to do anything to live a long and fruitful life, free of disease and medication? Wouldn't you want to know what you could do to help yourself, even if your own doctor did not have faith that you would do it?

(By the way, there are lots of doctors who do have faith in your ability to take control of your own health, and studies show this can make a difference in your health outcome. Go to one of them if possible! You will find a list at www.pcrm.org.)

I'll tell you what one decidedly UNaverage American did. After Bill Clinton's 2004 emergency heart surgery, he went to those doctors who had seen dramatic results treating their patients through nutritional intervention. When he got down to choosing life or death, he chose life over McDonald's. You can too and I want to make sure that you have the information and resources to do so.

Imagine, G-d forbid, you were diagnosed with cancer tomorrow. Now imagine that your doctor told you that there is a diet you could eat that would dramatically increase your chances of survival and decrease your chances of a recurrence. Would you even have to think about sticking to that diet, even if it were a big shift for you? Compared to the toxic side effects of chemotherapy, how hard would it be to eat broccoli and avoid white bread? I say that knowing that there is no magic pill or food that cures cancer; and knowing how hard it is to eat well in our society, where even at the hardware store we're offered candy and soda at the checkout. The key to success here is to try to get rid of that "noise" and get back to basics: real food.

Unfortunately, simply eating broccoli can't entirely prevent or cure cancer. However, eating a healthy, plant based diet with plenty of cruciferous vegetables can actually make a big difference in your chances of getting cancer and cancer survival (see the cancer section of this chapter for more information).

Diet affects pretty much everything about how well our bodies work and what diseases we do and don't experience. It is not just about disease. Our diet also affects our cognitive abilities, sex life, ability to procreate, and the quantity and quality of our lives.

Eating a diet of real food, rather than the processed junk we are offered hundreds of times a day through advertisements, marketing, and physical proximity, will improve your health now and for the future. Who wants to get started?

My mom always told me it was a lucky accident that I happened to be born in the United States, where we enjoy a standard of living and freedom most of the world can only dream about. Unfortunately, our quality of life is currently at risk. We are free but we are also free to eat ourselves to death; and many people do.

According to an annual survey conducted by the Organization for Economic Co-operation and Development (OECD), of its 34 member developed nations, the United States is the most obese, at 36.5 percent of the population.[xli]

Keep in mind that this number (over one third) covers obesity, not overweight. According to the Centers for Disease Control, approximately 70 percent of the United States population is overweight or obese. That means that only 1 in three people in the United States maintains a healthy weight.

In addition, according to the OECD study, 25 of the 34 nations have a higher life expectancy than the U.S. The U.S. spends the most on total health care compared with other nations, 17.7 percent of its Gross Domestic Product (almost 50 percent more than the next highest nation). The authors attribute the study findings to poor dietary habits, lack of exercise, a fragmented health care system, and a high uninsured population. This is not the United States in which my mom told me I was lucky to be born. This is the United States of relentless marketing and advertising for processed foods.

The United States where "moderation" is the mantra from health practitioners, has some of the highest rates of infant mortality, dementia, diabetes, and death from heart disease among developed nations.

Moderation may work for some, but obviously not for most. Keeping the taste of addictive foods in our mouths and our brains only makes us want more. If you could cut your cholesterol 100 points through diet alone (and you can), wouldn't you choose to make yourself "heart-attack proof"?

Although moderation sounds like a perfectly sane idea, the moderation of a horrible diet still doesn't equal a healthy one!

You deserve to know how diet affects some of our most common health issues and how YOU HAVE THE POWER TO CHANGE YOUR HEALTH AND QUALITY OF LIFE.

Here's more information about the dietary effects on the following:

1. Weight
2. Heart disease
3. Cancer
4. Diabetes
5. Stroke
6. Cognitive abilities and decline/Alzheimer's/dementia/memory
7. Quality and quantity of life
8. Sex and fertility

You will notice that many of the conditions and diseases discussed in this book are inter-related. So, while I tease out specifics for each category and in each chapter, it is hard to completely isolate the medical effects of the Standard American Diet (SAD).

WEIGHT

Vegan Diets Associated with Lower Weights

People who follow vegan diets weigh less. Among 71,751 participants enrolled in the highly respected Adventist Health Study 2 for five years, levels of BMI and rates of obesity went up as animal product intake increased.[xlii] Those categorized as vegan (eating animal products less than once per month), consumed the most beta-carotene, fiber, potassium, and magnesium; had the lowest average body mass index; and had the lowest prevalence of obesity.

Non-vegetarians (eating animal products without restriction) ate the most saturated fat and the least fiber, compared with the vegan group.

Plant Based Diets Better for Weight Loss

Another study followed 63 obese and overweight adults on an eight-week weight-loss program. Using the same dietary categories as above, findings presented at the Obesity Society's annual conference found that a plant based diet leads to more weight loss.

For each regimen, researchers encouraged low-fat, low-glycemic index foods without caloric restrictions and offered support from weekly classes.

Participants following the plant based diets lost the most weight, compared with those following the non-vegetarian diets. The researchers suggest plant based diets may work better for weight loss, **because they do not focus on portion control or calorie counting.**[xliii]

Why weight matters

Obesity contributes to sleep-breathing disorders, Type 2 diabetes, heart disease, asthma, and cancer. Is it possible that obesity will replace malnutrition and infectious diseases as the biggest reason for poor health?

Even being moderately overweight contributes to greater morbidity and mortality, with intra-abdominal fat its own specific danger.[xliv]

Obesity is an independent risk factor for cardiovascular disease for adults[xlv]

In children, obesity contributes to enlarged and thickened hearts, elevated cholesterol, blood pressure and sugar levels.[xlvi]

Obesity also contributes to asthma-related inflammation of the lungs and airways and is thought to be a major contributor to the doubled prevalence of asthma between 1986 and 2005. Almost 10 percent of children now have asthma. [xlvii]

Even if your child is not overweight, you should still be concerned about their level of nutrition and how much sugar they are ingesting, particularly sugar-sweetened beverages, as they increase the risk for asthma. Eating well has the opposite effect, lowering your child's risk for asthma (and other chronic diseases).[xlviii]
For children, weight loss can improve asthma symptoms and for adults, even a single fast-food meal will result in increased airway inflammation. [xlix]

HEART DISEASE
Unfortunately, cardiovascular disease is responsible for one out of every 3 deaths in the United States. Fortunately, it is entirely preventable and reversible.

The prevalence of heart disease in U.S. adults appears inevitable in light of the following figures:

33% have hypertension

13.8% have total cholesterol above 240 mg/dl[l]

11.3% of U.S. adults have diabetes[li] and

68.8% of U.S. adults are overweight or obese[lii]

Dr Fuhrman says, "If you eat the standard western diet that most people eat in the modern world, you will surely develop heart disease and may die from it."[liii]

Here is some information I found surprising and you may too:

Surgery and prescription drugs do not cure heart disease.

Numerous studies have found that angioplasty and bypass surgery, among other surgical interventions commonly used to treat heart disease, have the same results as prescription drugs, coupled with moderate lifestyle changes.[liv] Invasive surgery does not equal fewer heart attacks or a longer life.

Surgical interventions treat one blocked portion of a blood vessel. In the meantime, the rest of the arteries continue to narrow with heart attack and stroke causing plaque.

Cholesterol-lowering statin drugs are known to increase the risk of:

- Diabetes
- Impaired muscle function
- Cataracts
- Liver dysfunction
- Kidney injury[lv]

Blood pressure-lowering medications are associated with:

- Persistent cough
- Increased risk of diabetes
- Increased likelihood of stroke
- Increased risk of heart attack
- Increased risk of breast and lung cancer[lvi]

The risk associated with these treatments is unacceptable when there is a safe, effective alternative — excellent nutrition and exercise — that can actually reverse heart disease and obliterate the needs for risky and even futile medical care.
– Dr. Joel Fuhrman[lvii]

Here are two more reasons to address heart disease using nutrition.

Byproduct of Eating Animal Products Leads to Heart Failure
According to a study published in the *Journal of the American College of Cardiology*, a higher level of the chemical produced when the body digests foods like organ meat, red meat and eggs, resulted in a 3.4 fold increase in the risk of dying, compared to those with the lowest levels of the chemical, trimethylamine N-oxide (TMAO). The researchers followed 720 patients who had previously been treated for heart failure, for five years. [lviii]

Statin Users Gain Weight

According to a recently published study, partially titled, "Gluttony in the time of statins?", patients who take cholesterol-lowering drugs gain more weight and eat more fat and calories, than those not taking the medication.[lix]

For those placed on statins, over the course of ten years:

- Calorie intake increased 9.6 percent
- Fat intake increased 14.4 percent
- Weight increased more than in those not on medications

A number of doctors have concluded that a false sense of security has replaced nutritional improvements.

CANCER

The China Study and many others show that there is a direct link between the amount of animal protein consumed and cancer risk.

There are also specific foods that affect the risk of specific cancers. For instance, according to recent studies:

Eating beans, peas, or lentils more than 2 times per week can decrease your chance of colon cancer by 50 percent. Considering that colon cancer is the second most deadly cancer, this is a pretty easy way to lower your cancer risk.[lx]

Meat

The World Cancer Research Fund says the link between processed meat and cancer is so strong that it should be avoided completely. Eating processed meat is linked with a 44 percent increased risk of death and red meat with a 14 percent increased risk of death.[lxi]

Colorectal cancer survivors who consume the most red or processed meat are more likely to die over a 7.5-year follow-up, compared with those who eat the least, according to a new study from the American Cancer Society. Researchers found a 29 percent higher risk of death from all causes and a 63 percent higher risk of death from heart disease for those who consumed the most red and processed meat before diagnosis, compared with those who ate the least.[lxii]

Fish and Wine

A diet abundant in fish and wine increased the risk of estrogen and progesterone receptor positive breast cancer by 29 percent.[lxiii]

Plants

In a recent study of California teachers, following a plant based diet cut the risk of breast cancer by 15 percent, compared to those who did not eat many fruits and vegetables.[lxiv]

Cruciferous vegetables lower cancer risk by 40 percent

Dr. Fuhrman plotted cancer incidence in 25 countries against unrefined plant food intake and found that as vegetables, beans, and fruit consumption goes UP 20 percent in a population, cancer rates typically DROP 20 percent. However, as cruciferous vegetable intake increases 20 percent, cancer rates drop 40 percent! That means they are TWICE as effective as other fruits and vegetables at lowering cancer risk.[lxv]

Dairy

According to the Harvard Physicians' Health Study, men who consume more than 2.5 servings of dairy per day have a 34 percent increased risk of prostate cancer, compared to men who consume less than half a serving per day.

In the Health Professionals Follow-Up Study, men who consume two servings of milk per day show a 60 percent higher risk of prostate cancer compared to men who consume zero servings per day.

DIABETES

A low-saturated-fat diet improves insulin function and eating a low-saturated-fat, high-fiber diet helps with insulin sensitivity.[lxvi]

High-Fat, High-Protein Diets Linked to Type 2 Diabetes

A diet high in protein and fat and low in carbohydrate may increase the risk of developing Type 2 diabetes. In one study, women with diets high in meat and low in carbohydrates and plant foods, had a 56 percent greater chance of developing diabetes, compared with those eating diets high in fruits and vegetables.[lxvii]

Milk intake linked to Type 1 Diabetes

A number of studies suggest that an increased intake of milk as a child can lead to a higher risk of Type 1 diabetes.[lxviii]

STROKE

Most of us have, unfortunately, seen at least one family member or friend debilitated by a stroke. That is, if they survived at all.

A stroke can occur when:

- A blood clot prevents blood flow to brain, resulting in the abrupt death of brain cells.
- Plaque material or pieces of blood clots travel to the brain.
- High blood pressure leads to bleeding from a broken blood vessel in the brain.[lxix]

Some risk factors for stroke have nothing to do with diet, like taking birth control pills and smoking.

The risk factors for stroke that *are* caused by a poor diet include:

- Atherosclerotic plaque/hardening of the arteries
- Clots inside your blood vessels

- Decreased blood flow to the brain
- High blood pressure
- Diabetes

Blood pressure medication can prevent strokes but not heart attacks, meaning patients are still at a high risk of death from their high blood pressure.[lxx]

Homocysteine is an amino acid that increases after eating meat. High levels in the blood are a risk factor for heart disease, stroke and pulmonary embolism. High levels can be lowered by increasing folate and B vitamin intake through eating a variety of fruits and green leafy vegetables and taking a B12 supplement.

The good news is that a plant based diet can prevent both heart attacks and strokes, without the side effects or costs associated with prescription medicine.

COGNITIVE ABILITIES AND DECLINE/ALZHEIMERS/DEMENTIA/MEMORY

Ever feel sharper after a workout?

Ever feel foggy after eating a lot of fatty foods?

There is a reason for this. As mentioned previously, none of these health events occur in isolation. Lack of oxygen to the brain, caused by hardening and narrowing of the arteries, decreases blood flow to the brain and contributes to dementia.

A low-fat, low cholesterol diet keeps your brain healthy by providing open paths for oxygen to reach your brain. Exercise is another crucial way to increase the level of oxygen that reaches your brain.

Researchers from the longitudinal Chicago Health and Aging Project analyzed the diets of thousands of people over a number of years, and concluded that diet most definitely affects one's Alzheimer's risk.[lxxi]

Foods that increased Alzheimer's risk:

- Saturated "bad" fat—found in milk, cheese, and meat increases risk more than threefold.

- Trans fats, like those in doughnuts and snack cakes, increase risk fivefold.

Foods that reduced dementia risk by as much as 70 percent:

Foods rich in vitamin E, such as broccoli, almonds, walnuts, hazelnuts, pine nuts, pecans, pistachios, sunflower seeds, sesame seeds, and flaxseed.

Physicians Committee president Dr. Neal Barnard, compares the battle between clinicians and unhealthy food to the battle over tobacco a generation ago. He says that battle was won, but the current battle is over Alzheimer's-promoting foods that contain saturated and trans fats.

This is his call to action. "Research is rarely clean and unambiguous. But we potentially have the capabilities to prevent a disease that is poised to affect 100 million people worldwide by 2050. Why wait?"

PCRM's *Dietary Guidelines for Alzheimer's Prevention* recommends brain-healthy habits similar to those that prevent heart disease.

Dr. Barnard's recommendations to maximize brain-protection:

- Avoid the saturated and trans fats found in meats, dairy products, and snack foods.

- Base your diet on plant based foods.

- Add healthful sources of vitamin E, such as tofu, spinach and almonds.

- Combine this diet with physical exercise and avoid excess metals—such as iron and copper in multivitamins.

Here is a short list of Dr. Neil Barnard's Brain Protecting Foods:

Blueberries and grapes
Sweet potatoes
Green leafy vegetables
Beans and chickpeas

QUALITY AND QUANTITY OF LIFE

Red and Processed Meat Products Linked to Mortality

The consumption of red and processed meat products is associated with an increased risk of death.[lxxii]

Researchers found a 23 percent increase in mortality risk for those consuming the most processed meat.

Researchers found a 29 percent increased risk of death for those consuming the most total red meat, compared with those who consumed the least.

Diet Fuels Depression

Women who consume a diet defined as inflammatory, high in:

- Red meat
- Fish
- Sodas
- Refined grains

have a 41 percent higher risk for depression, compared with women who consume low amounts of these products.[lxxiii]

Osteoporosis

Americans are told by the dairy industry that we need more calcium and that it should be from dairy foods. In actuality, Americans consume too much calcium and from the wrong sources.

A three cup serving of raw, leafy greens provides the same amount of calcium (or more) as one cup of whole milk. In addition, only 32% of the calcium in the milk can be absorbed by the human body compared to about 50% for many green vegetables.[lxxiv] Greens also contain Vitamin K, which supports bone health.

According to a new study in the *British Medical Journal,* **milk is particularly dangerous for women, the group most targeted by dairy industry marketing.**

These are the results of drinking 3 cups of milk per day, compared to drinking 1 or less:

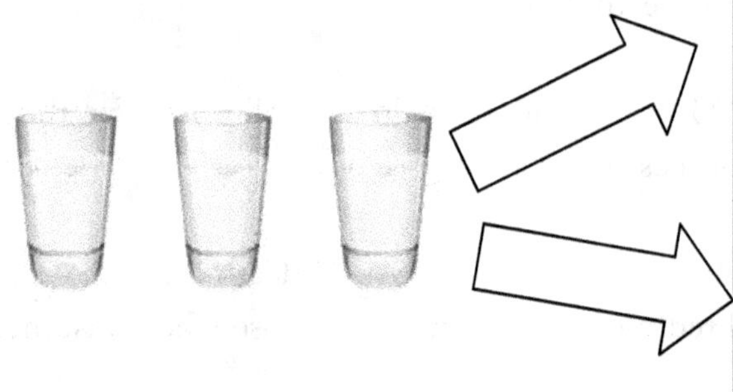

93 percent increased risk of dying, compared to women who drank less than one glass of milk per day.

60 percent increased risk of hip fracture and 16 percent increased risk for developing any bone fracture, compared to women who drank less than one glass of milk per day.

vs.

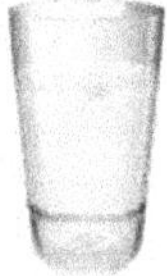

Additionally among women, for each glass of milk consumed, risk of dying from all causes increased by 15 percent, from heart disease by 15 percent, and from cancer by 7 percent.

In contrast, men had only a 10 percent increased risk of dying when consuming three or more glasses of milk per day, compared with those who drank less than one glass.[lxxv]

SEX AND FERTILITY

Sexual pleasure involves blood flow. The easier your blood flows, the more pleasure you can experience! The ease with which your blood flows is affected by your diet, physical activity and health conditions.

For instance, diabetes can cause vascular changes and nerve damage, impeding arousal and orgasm in both men and women.[lxxvi]

In addition, erectile dysfunction is often a sign of current or coming cardiac disease.[lxxvii]

- Men with only mild dysfunction face a significant extra risk of developing cardiovascular conditions in the future.

- As dysfunction increases, so do the signs of heart disease and the risk of earlier death.

The study's researchers found that the men with severe erectile dysfunction were:

- Eight times more likely to have heart failure
- 60 percent more likely to have heart disease
- Almost twice as likely to die of any cause

Physical activity and leanness are associated with maintenance of erectile function.

A recent study published in *The Journal of the American Medical Association*, looked at the effects of weight loss and increased physical activity on erectile function in men.[lxxviii]

About one third of the obese men with erectile dysfunction that lost weight and increased physical activity saw improvement in sexual function.

Even without dietary changes, research shows that exercise can help reverse diabetes symptoms and increase blood flow throughout the body, including the regions that provide sexual pleasure and function. In addition, exercise can increase the production of sex hormones, such as testosterone.

Fertility

An unhealthy lifestyle can also prevent or delay pregnancy. According to a study led by the National Institute of Child Health and Human Development, couples with higher total cholesterol levels showed lower pregnancy rates or took longer to become pregnant, compared with those who had lower levels.[lxxix]

Sperm Quality

Processed meat products may lower sperm quality, according to an abstract presented by Harvard at the American Society for Reproductive Medicine's annual conference.

Men who were having reproductive difficulties reported higher intakes of processed meat products (more than one-third of a serving per day) saw more abnormalities in sperm count, size, and shape, compared with men who ate less.[lxxx]

The Future

Susan Levin, M.S., R.D., C.S.S.D., director of nutrition education at PCRM, told Clinicians at the 2014 International Nutrition and the Brain Summit that they need to set a good example. "Nutrition and lifestyle changes should be at the core of 'conventional' medical practice. Medications should serve as 'alternative' medicine, when nutrition and lifestyle changes are not enough."

"The unfortunate diet habits baby boomers developed in the 70s and 80s are now bearing their fruit," says Dr. Barnard.

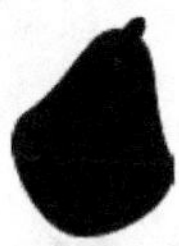

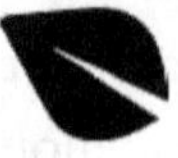

"Turn on a TV. Half of the commercials are for high-fat snacks and junk food. The other half are for medications to reverse the effects of those foods."

-Dr. Neal Barnard

4

10 STEPS TO A HEALTHY DIET FOR A LIFETIME

Even with everything you have to do, your children's health and well-being is at the top of your priority list each and every day. When the "6 o'clock scramble" comes along, you need easy and healthy ideas. You need guidelines that help you, not make you feel like you are not doing enough (of whatever it is you are supposed to be doing). You need a balance between laborious intensive preparation and giving your kids macaroni and cheese *every* night.

You can't be an expert at everything. I happen to have a passionate interest in health and nutrition. I have read dozens of books and experimented on myself and my own family. Although I recommend a vegan diet, I am going to keep reminding you that vegan doesn't always equal healthy.

It is as much about what you do eat as what you don't eat and most people don't know what to eat.

That is why I wrote a whole book for you! I want the good food to crowd out the non-nutritive food.

If you could choose (and you can) would you make your diet about abundance or restriction? I am here to provide you with the abundance option. People always *inform* me that, as a vegan, I must feel so limited in my food choices. I say, it's the opposite. Taking out the usual pizza and fries, meat and potatoes meals makes me expand my creativity in the kitchen. I eat adventurously and with a lot more variety than most people. I always feel like the possibilities are endless. Cutting out meat and dairy just means I expand in other places, like fruits, vegetables, legumes, seeds, nuts, twigs, stones...Okay, those last two were just to see if you were paying attention!

The bottom line is this:
Constantly looking to add more nutritious food to your meals is sustainable and will lead to a healthy life and a healthy weight. Simply slashing calories, portion size and all carbohydrates will lead you to a rollercoaster of shame, unwanted pounds and feeling like crap.

Ten Steps to a Healthy Diet for a Lifetime

1. Sculpt a healthy lifestyle, one layer at a time

I have been thinking for a long time about the right metaphor for the multi-layered and patient approach that it takes to improve your lifestyle and dietary habits - in a sustainable way.

Think of your health as a plaster sculpture of your own design. First, decide what type of sculpture you want to make. In other words, what type of physical and mental physique do you want to create?

Next, figure out how to sculpt that physique. (See steps 2-10!)

Once you know the necessary path to creating your sculpture (the new you), add the first layer of plaster (step 2) and wait for it to dry.

When you are sure it is hard enough, and you have absorbed that step into your daily routine, move onto the next layer of plaster (step 3).

Wait for that layer to set. Then move on to the next step until you have molded all 10 layers of plaster and your life is on the right path.

Keep reading, layering the changes, and waiting until each healthy habit is set to move forward. Although it may not sound like the quick fix you are looking for, that is the recipe for lasting change, health and happiness. Isn't that better than living in fear that all of your weight loss will come back the second you get to your goal weight?

Other authors make their money by promising quick weight loss. You may very well experience that when you follow my recommendations, but that isn't the focus here. I want you to feel physically and mentally energetic and happy because you have a plan for yourself and your family. I do promise happiness and empowerment – the type of lasting happiness that comes with being clear on what you want for yourself and your family and making it happen.

I don't want you to "white knuckle" it. Allow the changes you are making to empower you and your family. You *can* control how you feel today and your future quality of life.

Change your eating habits and you *will* feel leaner and like a new person in one day. Is that quick enough? Even better, you and your children will enjoy this feeling of good health together, for a long time.

2. Focus on nutrition, not calories

While most grown-ups want to focus on eating less food and fewer calories to lose weight, that doesn't set them up for a mindset of abundance and permanent change.

The traditional focus on calories in, calories out doesn't work for a number of reasons. First of all, it is very difficult to estimate calories correctly. Second, healthy plant based foods like vegetables, fruit and legumes naturally contain fewer calories and can be eaten in greater quantities than processed meat, white flour foods and sugar.

Finally, as you read in Chapter 2, health and weight are the sum of more than total calories. Calories from healthy carbohydrates metabolize faster than the calories from meat and sugar. They're also more satiating and energizing. You will feel full faster and longer.

Focus on eating more at each meal, instead of eating all day!

The key here is to remember we are talking about individual meals and not one long day of grazing.

Humans need to feel like we've truly eaten in order to be satisfied. That is one reason that sitting down to eat without distractions helps us feel full quicker. We realize that we've eaten both physically and mentally more than when we graze standing at the counter or snack while watching TV. In addition, while cooking dinner, we can easily taste and snack on a meal's worth of calories but not feel like we ate at all.

A larger serving of plant based food will also be more satisfying to your brain, belly and body. Chewing and swallowing a big plate of food tells us that we've eaten and we are ready to do something else. It helps prevent the day from being one long meal.

Meal planning helps. It will give you so much clarity into what you are really eating when you can say, I had x for breakfast, x for lunch and x for dinner. Even better, write down your daily (or weekly) menu and post it in your kitchen.

For your children, it is not emotionally healthy to focus on counting calories and limiting food. The healthiest way to approach the subject of food with children is to focus on what to eat, not how much. Once they're eating real food and you address any emotional eating issues, their portions will control themselves.

Parents know that eating well is also about long-term health, but children can't comprehend the long-term benefits of a healthy diet. Instead, focus on the positive effects of healthy foods on their mood and energy for walking around the mall with their friends, making it through the school day or going on a family ski trip.

Children who eat the right foods will feel the immediate results of their good health.

Just like grown-ups, they will see that the foods they once ate on a regular basis now make them feel yucky and lethargic. In addition, they probably won't even taste good. In fact, my husband said he has felt this transformation for himself.

My kids are so used to homemade cookies (see the oatmeal banana chocolate chip recipe in *The Healthy Family, Healthy You Cookbook*!) made with pure ingredients, that the other day, when someone gave them store-bought preservative-filled chocolate chip cookies, they rejected them. The kids (and my husband) thought they were "gross." I was such a proud mama!

3. Become your own ideal child

Imagine how you would want your children to eat in an ideal world. Now, start working towards eating that way yourself.

We can't tell our children to enjoy a frozen banana for dessert while we eat a pan of brownies. This can be a curse and a blessing. I choose to focus on the blessing part. If you want your kids to eat 5 fruits and vegetables a day, you need to show them how to do it by showing them *how* **you** *do it* (and, just for the record, adults need closer to 10 servings per day, rather than 5. Eating plants for your protein makes it much easier to get there). Surrounded by fast food advertisements, they may think it's "weird" to eat real food. The more they see you eat real food and experience eating it themselves, the better. The more real food they eat, the worse they'll feel when they eat junk.

You can't create a clear dichotomy between real and junk food unless your house is an oasis of healthy options.

Don't allow foods in your house that you don't actually want your children to eat. This one action will eliminate most snack and meal time battles.

Remember the following:

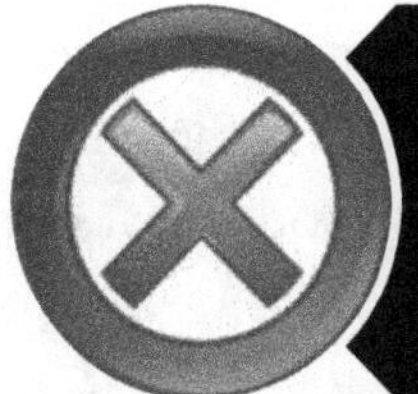

Kids don't need store-bought artificial processed cookies to survive. If they "need" a treat, or you want to give them one for a special occassion, they'll do just fine on healthier homemade cookies and desserts.

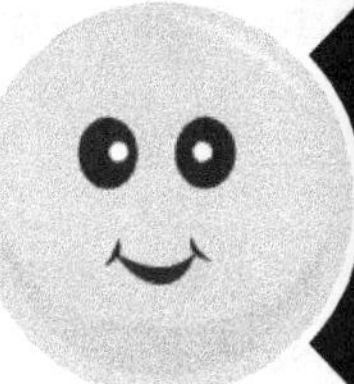

Our taste buds become accustomed to what we eat and start to crave those specific foods. Simply remembering that can help keep you motivated to feed your children well, despite their initial protests.

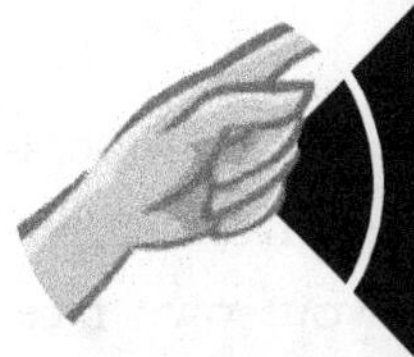

You are the parent, not the corporation. The corporation is in it for the money, not your child's future health and well-being. That's your job and you can do it!

4. Develop strategies for your own household

A friend of mine said she knows the best day of he week to try to get her daughter to try new fruits and vegetables. When she comes home from baseball she is starving. She'll eat almost anything she is given.

When I pick up the kids from school I'll often specifically leave any drinks at home and bring a bowl of cut-up watermelon or cantaloupe. Without other choices, they eat it up and realize how refreshing the fruit tastes. It also quenches their thirst, encouraging them to eat more fruit and stop begging me for the juice boxes I won't bring them.

After this healthy snack, they're less hungry if they're going to an activity where they see more food choices, most of which I do not want them to eat. An example is the numerous ice cream machines we encounter at the community center we go to for *healthy exercise* activities. It just never ends. Everyone is trying to shove junk food down our throats.

To remind yourself of how important your job is, think of what they would eat if left to their own devices and outside influences: pizza, fries, and ice cream for every meal.

The other day we stopped for gas and I heard from the loudspeaker the equivalent of, "You know you want it. Come inside for super cheap, super delicious mouth-watering food and sweet soda."

Even Home Depot has candy and soda at the cash register. My kids go with my husband to pick up something and it becomes an occasion for them to beg for candy! It's hard to catch a break from corporations pushing soda, candy and other junk food in your own face. How much harder must it be for your children, as they are specifically targeted as customers who can develop life-long loyalties to specific brands of junk food?

They also believe commercials without question. My daughter will repeat them to me verbatim, with the same intonation as the commercial's narrator, but with her own emotion in it. "They make the perfect snack!" she says to me about a food she has seen on a specific commercial.

Instead of believing these commercial messages, you want to help them develop a life-long belief in and affinity for real food. It is never too late for you, your kids or anyone in your circle of family and friends. So why wait?

Be a rebel. Don't let it in! Don't let your kids become one of an increasing number of teenagers showing signs of heart disease and Type 2 diabetes.

It will also help you to set a good example for your children if you understand why it is hard for you (and them) to resist the call of certain foods.

5. Understand food cravings and addictive foods

It is important to know that there are real reasons why it feels so overwhelming and difficult to change your diet permanently. Michael Moss's book, "Salt, Sugar, Fat,"[lxxxi] illuminated two important points for me:

First, I am a constant target of advertisers trying to sabotage any healthy choices I intend to make. Sometimes they do this by trying to convince me that their product is a healthy choice, even if it is not; or by putting little cakes and whipped cream next to the strawberries, to cement my association that eating strawberries means eating strawberry short cake. Even the produce aisle is no longer a safe, temptation free zone.

Second, there is a reason I want to eat a whole bag of chips or pint of ice cream, instead of a "serving." Someone in a laboratory spent a long time testing out different chemical combinations to make sure my brain will light up with pleasure, my stomach won't register that I have eaten and I'll want more and more.

Sometimes I'll look at something processed and just not want to go there. I know the temporary pleasure it will bring me. However, I don't want to then feel bad physically and mentally after I wasn't able to eat just a little bit - or even if I was - I was miserable while I controlled myself. Knowing it is not my fault that I want to keep eating junk food removes guilt and self-blame. I know that for a lot of people this cycle feeds their overeating. Processed food is like any addiction: It takes more and more to get the same feelings of bliss. Afterwards you feel badly about your lack of self-control. This low self-esteem leads to feelings of hopelessness and the whole cycle starts all over again.

Step out of this cycle by avoiding these foods and enjoy feeling empowered, rather than helpless, in the face of a bag of chips or cookies.

6. Focus on quality, not quantity

What to eat.

When choosing your food, focus on the micronutrient to calorie ratio. For example, 1 cup of raspberries contains less than 6 grams of natural sugar, along with 64 calories, 8 grams of fiber and countless disease-fighting micronutrients (vitamins, minerals and phytochemicals you can only get from real food). Your average 1 cup of candy contains 652 calories, 129 grams of added sugar, no fiber and no nutrition. Sometimes, just looking at something like that intellectually can give me an aha moment and help me easily make the right choice.

For nutrient density made easy, I try to follow Dr. Joel Fuhrman's recommendations:

- Make a gigantic salad the main dish of at least 1 meal per day.

- Eat lots of onions, mushrooms and beans. (Add them to a dish you are already making).

- Have your blood tested for vitamin deficiencies. Most people need to take a Vitamin D supplement and omega-3 fatty acid supplement.

- Eat two servings per day of steamed leafy greens.

- Use fruit to satisfy your natural sweet tooth.

- Avoid fake and processed foods.

Even if I cover half of these recommendations each day, I am in a much better place than I might be if I did not make any intentional efforts.

Dr. Fuhrman, specifically recommends eating the following foods to prevent and treat most diseases. It's simple, yet comprehensive, which is why I give it to you now:

- Greens
- Beans
- Onions
- Mushrooms
- Berries
- Pomegranates
- Seeds and nuts
- Cruciferous vegetables

Benefits include boosting the immune system, preventing diabetes and cancer and increasing rates of cancer survival.[lxxxii]

I don't know about you, but I know I used to spend forever reading labels on the back of protein bars. I wanted to balance sugar and fat with fiber and protein. Now I never touch those things, except an occasional Lara or Kind bar. I am laughing at myself right now, remembering how I used to work out with a personal trainer in the morning and then I would be so hungry I'd end up eating two Cliff or Balance bars. Yeah, not so helpful for weight control! Just another example of why real food is always the best choice.

What if you found a bar that had 100 calories, zero fat, zero sugar, 7 grams of fiber, and 8 grams of protein? Oh and it costs 50 cents. You know what that is? That is the information for the half cup of beans I added to my lunch salad today.

Cruciferous vegetables

Cruciferous vegetables are the rock stars of cancer prevention.[lxxxiii] Eating 20% more can lower your cancer risk by 40%.[lxxxiv] You don't have to ask me twice. I'm there!

Here's a quick list of cruciferous vegetables:

arugula
bok choy
broccoli
broccoli rabe
broccolini
Brussels sprouts
cabbage
cauliflower
collards
horseradish
kale
kohlrabi
mustard greens
radish
red cabbage
rutabaga
turnips
turnip greens
watercress

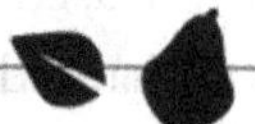

Use cauliflower as your new "cream" soup base (see Resources for additional, related ideas). Add mandolin-cut radishes and arugula to your salad. Roast Brussels sprouts. Keep frozen broccoli around for a quick side dish or addition to your black bean pasta. Slip kale, mustard greens or watercress into your green smoothie. Make mayo-less coleslaw with red and green cabbage. Add bok choy to your stir fry or green smoothie.

Fiber-filled foods

Fiber prevents:

- Heart Disease
- Colon Cancer
- Type 2 Diabetes

Every 10 grams of fiber consumed daily provides a 12% reduction in colon cancer risk.[lxxxv] It does this by reducing the contact between dietary carcinogens and intestinal cells by increasing stool volume and accelerating transit time.[lxxxvi]

Fiber also lowers cholesterol, preventing heart disease.

Foods that are naturally high fiber, such as beans and whole grains, come with additional benefits as well, including beneficial probiotics, protein and phytochemicals. Fiber lowers insulin resistance, thus preventing Type 2 Diabetes. In addition, high fiber beans are the best source of starch for diabetics.[lxxxvii]

According to Registered Dietician Joy Bauer, nutrition and health expert for NBC's *Today* show, "Beans are a winning combination of high-quality carbohydrates, lean protein, and soluble fiber that helps stabilize your body's blood-sugar levels and keeps hunger in check. Beans are also inexpensive, versatile, and virtually fat-free."[lxxxviii]

7. Subtract animal protein

As I have shown, dairy and meat cause cancer, heart disease and diabetes. Do you really need additional reasons to avoid them? When there are protein-filled foods that also contain disease-fighting phytochemicals (such as beans), why would you choose the protein source that causes cancer instead of fights it? Yeah, I don't know either! Also, keep in mind that the more animal protein people eat, the more disease-promoting saturated fat and the fewer disease-fighting plants they consume.

Animal protein=more fat, more disease.

Plant protein=less fat, less disease.

I understand that some people would really miss the flavor of meat (and poultry, etc…) and that cutting it out entirely does not feel like an option for them. In that case, there are other strategies.

1. Use meat as a flavor agent more instead of as the main dish.

2. Choose meat that is humanely raised without antibiotics and hormones. The cost of this alone will help you cut down your meat consumption considerably!

3. Consider meat a treat for special occasions, rather than the basis for most meals.

8. Eat the right fat and avoid the wrong fat

Here are my rules about fat:

1. Don't eat food items that are unnaturally and artificially fat-free, like fat-free cookies and potato chips.

2. Keep oils to a minimum, including choices that most consider healthy, like olive oil and grapeseed oil. At the end of the day, the good stuff in the food is not in the oil. Just because olive oil is better for you than something like peanut oil, doesn't mean you should go to town. What about the Mediterranean diet? Some assert that the reason the Mediterranean diet has proven healthy is because of the high content of tomatoes, walnuts and beans, not olive oil.

All oil contains 120 calories per tablespoon and is almost instantly converted to body fat. Almost all the processed food that Americans eat contains some sort of vegetable oil, providing our bodies with a quick injection of fat, without much nutrition.

Yes, we need fat to function, but we don't need saturated fat or pure fat in the form of oils. Americans high consumption of oils simply leads to obesity and chronic disease.

Save your fat for foods that provide you with "good fat," that which contain omega 3 and omega 6, and have real health benefits. Yes, fish contains healthy fat, but it also contains unhealthy fat, cholesterol and numerous environmental pollutants.

Do eat plant foods that naturally contain healthy fat, such as nuts, seeds and avocados. If you need to watch your weight, keep to ¼ of an avocado, 1 Tablespoon nuts, and 1 teaspoon seeds per day.

9. Remember, "White ain't right!"

Here are the facts. White bread, white rice and white potatoes are what are called high glycemic foods. This means they raise blood glucose levels quickly in comparison to low glycemic foods, such as unprocessed grains with their fiber and nutrients still intact. Eating high glycemic load foods is associated with cancer, heart disease, insulin resistance, Type 2 diabetes and weight gain.

Refined "white" bread and rice are stripped of the healthy fiber and micronutrients. What do you end up with? Foods with lots of calories that raise your blood sugar, promote diabetes, don't keep you full and don't contain much nutrition.

Refined grain consumption is associated with an increased risk of both colon and breast cancer.[lxxxix]

If you aren't accustomed to eating whole grains, here are a few suggestions:

- Brown and wild rice (serve with tofu and veggies)
- Wheat berries (great in salads)
- Barley (use it to thicken soups or as a pilaf with veggies)
- Quinoa (eat it hot like a pilaf, add it to your salad or make it into its own cold salad)
- Old fashioned oats (add pomegranate juice to them the night before for a quick and sweet, but added-sugar-free treat in the morning)
- You can also choose 100% whole grain bread and pasta. You will find information about bean and quinoa pastas in the Resources section. Those are even better choices than whole wheat pasta.

Buy grains that you can cook in water, such as wheat berries, quinoa and barley. Most processed grains, such as cereals, crackers and breads are dry cooked and can form a toxin called acrylamide in the browning process. High acrylamide intake is associated with several cancers."[xc]

In addition, you should know that whole grain pastry flour is ground so fine that it actually has a high glycemic index, taking away some of the benefit of the whole grain. Many studies have linked foods with a high glycemic index to an increased risk of colorectal cancers.[xci]

Carbohydrates are not your enemy! You will find something called 'resistant starch' in rolled oats, peas, beans and lentils.

Similar to fiber, resistant starch is a carbohydrate that fuels the growth of healthy bacteria in the gut, which have a number of anti-cancer effects.[xcii]

To reduce your intake of acrylamides and refined grains, try to replace some of your breads and pastas with low glycemic, high nutrient and high fiber beans, lentils, squash and sweet potatoes. Studies show that eating legumes, such as beans, peas or lentils, at least twice a week, can decrease colon cancer risk by 50%.[xciii]

10. Beat the sweet

By now, you probably know that sugar is bad for you. Sugar contributes to weight gain, heart disease, diabetes and cancer. There are several reasons why it's not so simple to avoid it.
It is addictive. Recent studies have shown that sugar lights up the same bliss points in our brain as cocaine!

It is in almost everything we buy in a package or can. In addition, manufacturers find ways to disguise when sugar is the most plentiful ingredient in their product. If they put four different forms of sugar in the ingredients, they are all listed separately, even if, together, they would make sugar the number one ingredient.

Because sugar is added to everything around us, our taste buds have become accustomed to it and real food no longer tastes good. For instance, when your baby first ate oatmeal, she probably ate happily without demanding that you sweeten it. Now, if your children are like most American kids, if it doesn't have maple brown sugar flavoring or little sugar-covered dinosaurs in it, they think its "gross."

If you internalize one idea from this chapter, make it this:

Don't be afraid to be different.

Dr. Fuhrman calls this way of eating being a "nutritarian." I was calling it "nutrarian" by accident, for years. That is because the word always reminds me of contrarian. Contrary to popular belief, you don't have to be mentally and physically incapacitated at the end of your life. Contrary to popular belief, it won't ruin your life to eat in a healthful manner. Quite the opposite, in fact.

Take charge now for short and long-term health benefits galore.

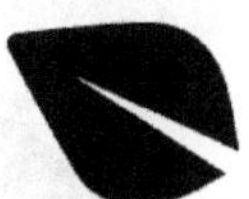

You can choose health (which = happiness) now.

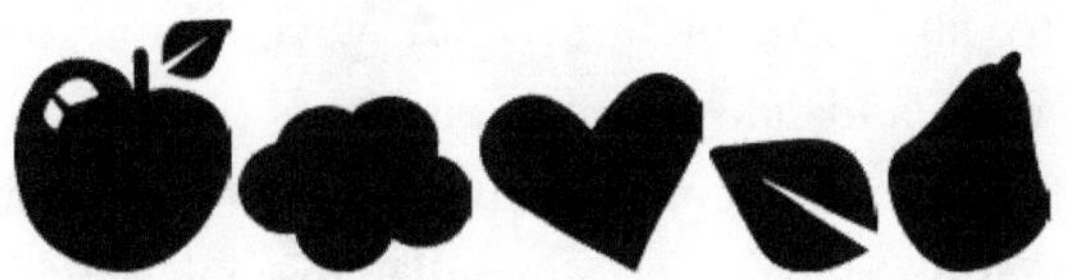

10 TOOLS TO CREATE A HEALTHY FAMILY FOR LIFE

Tool #1: Pick your battles

We all have plans for how our children will eat. The other parents will drool with jealousy over the varied and sophisticated palate of our little ones. They'll run around the playground clutching carrot and celery sticks and turn their nose up at white bread. This works for a while, until your child leaves the house. Then it's all over.

In reality, our kids' diets are out of our control much of the time. Even when we pack their lunches for daycare, camp, and preschool, they're often provided with snacks. Schools are responsive and understanding to allergen concerns. But what about food coloring, white flour, sugar, and salt? At my daughter's preschool, parents take turns buying snacks for the week. They give us a list that includes apples, bananas, and grapes. It also includes pretzels, cheese, and crackers.

I always buy whole wheat options when I buy the snack (although my husband does not), just as I would for my house. If I asked the other parents to do that, would I be laughed at? I simply don't want my child eating pretzels and crackers made of white flour, hydrogenated oil, sugar, and salt. Instead of preventing her from eating what other parents send in, I make it my goal to get anything and everything good in her when she's home.

When my sister started her son (child #1) at a prestigious daycare, she challenged the cheap, bulk, empty-carb snacks they serve, such as Ritz-type crackers. In addition, she was adamant that her son only consume organic dairy. The daycare provides non-organic milk to the children. She felt so strongly about her son's health, she was willing to risk causing a stir. She provided all of his food for a long time. Once, she was about to reign herself in and let them give him their applesauce at snack time. Then she looked at it. High-fructose corn syrup. Does a 12-month-old need HFCS with his applesauce every day? I think not! She felt vindicated for being so vigilant but sad that applesauce could become a forbidden food.

But then…she had child #2. She decided the non-organic, but non-RSBT (added hormones) milk is okay for the one cup child #1 drinks at school and she allows him to eat the provided lunch (the vegetarian option). She still packs his snacks.(In fact, she takes turns making snacks with another mom and then the two kids share each week. Go teamwork!) At some point, we have to give ourselves a break and do what we can without totally sacrificing our sanity. Any lunch she doesn't have to pack or milk she doesn't have to send in makes her life a little bit easier. As parents, we have to pick and choose our battles.

My daughter had a terrific first summer at day camp. However, she came home every day bouncing off the walls and cranky at the same time. By my estimation, between Laffy Taffy, fruit roll ups, lollipops, popsicles, and cookies, camp provided the kids with three to five items a day with food coloring. It is the only reason I can think of that she went back to normal immediately after camp ended. I understand why a camp operating a high-quality, reasonably-priced program would keep kids happy with treats and try to save money on snacks by buying industrial bags of cookies, crackers, and pretzels; and let's not forget those awful popsicles that come in a number of nuclear colors and are practically free when you buy them by the case.

I did not want to seem ungrateful by questioning the camp, but I also did not want my daughter ingesting food coloring on a daily basis, not just for her behavior, but her health. Before her second summer at the camp another mom and I researched relatively affordable popsicles without food coloring and gave the information to the camp. They were quite willing to change the popsicles and add more snacks of pure, unadulterated fruit. In fact, they even invited me to lead a few "fruit funshops" with the kids, who loved it. They had a lot of other details on their plate and just had not thought about the popsicles. Next summer, I might work on popsicles without corn syrup. One thing at a time! But the food coloring…there was no way I could let that go.

We all have a lot on our plates. I am not unsympathetic to the powers that be at schools and camp. That is why I go to them with great intentions, a smile on my face and helpful suggestions. I am willing to put in some of the work to establish new systems. If you don't have the time, maybe there is another parent who does. There is always something that can be done. You don't have to accept the status quo or compromise your children's health.

Nutrition matters. It affects health, energy, behavior, sleep and learning. Think about how you'd feel physically and mentally if you lived on pizza and fries (you know, what your kids try to do). You don't want your kids to feel lethargic and yucky.

TOOL #2: Create goals around food and health

Create your goals and then take on each change as you feel ready. Think of the changes you want to make as layers. Remember your sculpture in Chapter 4? After one layer solidifies, you can add the next.

After you (and your partner, if relevant) come up with the guidelines, you can hold a family meeting so kids can give their input into the plans for implementation. Kids are more likely to go for a new change if they feel they had a hand in the planning and aren't simply being told what to do.

Here are some ideas to help you create your own. Even if you only come up with two items for each category, you are on your way to living an intentionally healthy life and planning one for your children.

Example goals around food and health

Eat 5 different fruits and vegetables per day.
Get more exercise.
Spend more time together as a family, without electronics.
Eat as few laboratory-created ingredients as possible.
Increase energy and health in all family members.

Use the worksheet found later in this chapter to record your own.

TOOL #3: Create 10 family health commandments

Here are some ideas.

1. We will eat dinner together, without electronics, 3x per week.
2. We will all write down the fruits and vegetables we've eaten until a habit of eating at least 5 per day is entrenched in our routines.
3. We will spend family time together while engaged in physical activity at least 1x per week.

4. We will commit to eating only (or mostly) non-processed grab and go snacks, such as homemade granola bars and apples.
5. We will not buy more than one food per week with artificial food coloring.
6.
7.
8.
9.
10.

TOOL #4: Create a plan for implementation

After you come up with the first two lists, you may want to consider a plan for implementation. Look at these examples and see if they inspire you.

Example plan for implementation

1. Look for opportunities for fun family time that involves physical activity. Fill out a family calendar with different opportunities, like family festivals, paddle boating or a special tour though public gardens.

2. Create a rainbow chart for each family member. Make five spaces on the black and white rainbow. Fill out each space with the name of the fruit or vegetable you ate with a marker of that color. For instance, use an orange marker for a pumpkin or butternut squash or purple for grapes and eggplant. Give everyone their own page for each week or month and that way everyone can review their progress and the variety they have eaten. Mom and Dad too! You can also tell your kids that this system will ensure that parents don't forget to give them credit for every fruit and vegetable eaten. They'll like that.

Here's a blank example:

Day 1 MOM

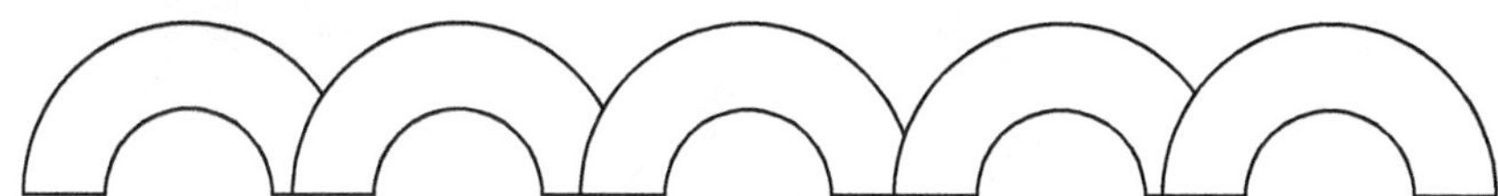

(Repeat for a total of 7 times for 1 week)

Day 1 DAD

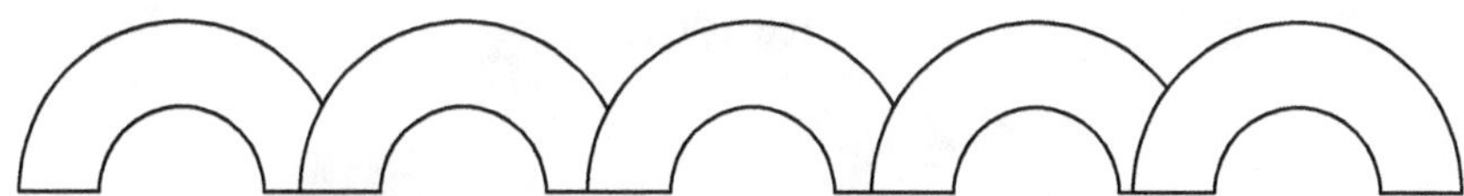

(Repeat for a total of 7 times for 1 week)

Etc....

3. Schedule your family dinners on agreed upon evenings that work with activities. Once everyone agrees on the nights, they'll know not to schedule other plans at that time.

4. Let each family member pick the fruit and vegetable for at least one dinner each week.

5. Etc...

Healthy Family, Healthy You

Sample blank family worksheet to photocopy and fill out

Goals around food and health

1.
2.
3.
4.
5.

10 Family Health Commandments

1.
2.
3.
4.
5.
6.
7.
8.
9.
10.

Plan for Implementation

1.
2.
3.
4.
5.

Do you know what your strongest weapon is in your fight against the artificial food industry? The one that spends billions/millions of dollars each year, coming up with the exact ratio of salt, sugar and fat to make sure you become addicted to their products; the one that uses more "food products" than food? Now, drumroll…

TOOL #5: Real Food. Shop for it. Eat it. Develop a taste for it.

You don't have to only shop the perimeter of the store. That advice is both too broad and too narrow. Shop the most at the entry, which is the produce section and where you should spend 75 percent of your grocery shopping time and budget. There are other valuable, and real, foods inside the perimeter. However, there are also worthless foods on the perimeter, like juices and yogurt with added sugar and food coloring or the aforementioned strawberry shortcake accoutrements smiling at you from the produce section.

It is okay to go into the middle of the store. You don't need to visit the cookie aisle… but you will want to buy oatmeal and other whole grains; frozen and canned fruits and vegetables; legumes (beans) and nuts.

You will even find some of the *Healthy Family, Healthy You* sanctioned "Fast Food" provided in this chapter. What is that you ask? The frozen section!

Just remember, you are still shopping for REAL WHOLE FOODS! No broccoli in cheese sauce or pre-sauced and seasoned rice and vegetables. Make sure you choose frozen fruits sans sugar. Look at the label. Never ever put it past food companies to put food coloring (and preservatives) in anything and everything. If it is super red, kids think it tastes better. Sometimes, they aren't familiar with the real taste or appearance of a particular food, especially fruits.

As an adult, you can probably conjure up the taste of a real banana vs. banana flavor, like that in taffy. What about real strawberry and orange vs. candy strawberry and candy orange? Just to give you one example: My favorite birthday cake; the one my twin sister and I insist my mom make every year; the one that she has made and shipped across the country several times; is simply called "orange cake." When I tell people its name, they look at me strangely, and I always have to explain it is made with, "real orange." I explain that it contains real orange oil, freshly grated orange zest and orange juice, mixed into a real vanilla cake recipe and topped with homemade frosting (with similar ingredients). After they have had it, they are simply stunned and want to be invited back for cake every year! (In case you are wondering, I have perfected making it vegan! Can't say healthy…but definitely healthier…).

The problem is that most of us, most especially children who are uber-targeted by marketing for these products, rarely have an opportunity to taste the real thing and remember how delicious and genuine it is. We often think of orange "flavor" before we think of the real thing.

When children cook with you and taste the individual ingredients, you are training their brains to recognize, appreciate, and prefer, the flavors in real food. The less processed, chemically-engineered foods people eat, the more their taste buds are able to actually taste real food. In addition, the more real food they eat, the more their taste buds are able to detect, and ultimately be repelled by, an artificial taste in processed foods.

People of every age can re-awaken their taste buds in only 1-3 weeks. I have done this for myself with Debby Amster, a health coach trained to teach Hale Sofia Schatz's[xciv] nutrition program. I was on the program for 10 days and ate only whole foods and eliminated all sweeteners. I was eating a sweet potato at every meal to keep me full and make up for the lack of bread or rice on the cleanse. At first I was putting pumpkin pie spice on my sweet potatoes each day. When that became too strong, I switched to cinnamon. Then, even the cinnamon was getting in the way of the full flavor of the sweet potato. This was in only one week!

Tool #6: Substitution is your strategy

Every person and every family has the top 20 food items they buy at the store and top 10 dishes they eat at home. The easiest way to eat well without thinking too hard is to simply substitute what you currently eat with new, healthier options.

For instance, what are the top foods you eat for breakfast, lunch, dinner and snacks? Use this page to fill in the categories below and then the substitute. I am not going to provide all of them for you because I don't have a recipe for every food on the planet, and I don't know what your favorites are currently. However, if I don't have it, someone else does. Sometimes I can tell you who and sometimes I can't. However, using the resource chapter (and my companion cookbook), I am confident you will find everything you need. In fact, filling out these resource worksheets will be a great opportunity for your whole family to work together and feel included in the process of becoming a healthier, happier family. If you are single, enlist a few friends you host for dinner parties or go out to eat with to brainstorm how you can support one another. You are also always welcome to ask me for help directly through my blog at www.healthyfamilyhealthyyou.com, through email at natasha@healthyfamilyhealthyyou.com, or on my Facebook page, https://www.facebook.com/NatashaRosenstockNadel.

If your favorite breakfast is blueberries and bananas in almond milk, you don't need to replace that one! Chances are though, that you will have others you can replace. As an example, I have filled out a sample worksheet using my own choices as an example.

Healthy Family, Healthy You

Top 5 breakfast items your family enjoys:

Item you eat now	Problem with it	New Solution	Benefits	New Recipe Source
Store-bought granola	Very high in fat	Homemade granola without added sugar and fat	Additional antioxidants from fruit Lower in sugar No added fat.	*Forks Over Knives Cookbook* by Del Sroufe, et
French toast	High in fat and sugar low in nutrients and whole grains	Whole-grain "Fronch Toast" and wild blueberry syrup	Skips animal products Adds antioxidants and whole grains Low in sugar	*The Post Pun Kitchen*, by Isa Chandra Moskowitz ("Fronch Toas is her term)
Store-bought muffins	High in fat, low in nutrients and whole grains	Chocolate Chip Banana Muffins	Skips animal products High in nutrients and antioxidants Lower in calories No added sugar	See recipe chapter
Chocolate milk shake	Added sugar, too high in calorie and saturated fats, not enough nutrients	Homemade smoothie	Lower in calories No added sugar or fat Higher in antioxidants	See recipe chapter

See the next chapter for more meal makeovers and recipes.

Come back to fill in these pages as you read through this book, and after, as you explore the suggested resources, including *The Healthy Family, Healthy You Cookbook.*

Please also make use of **The Magic 8 Authorized Fast Food List** in this chapter. Use it as an inspiration for quick meals and also photocopy it to keep on your fridge or with your grocery list.

I suggest you don't write in the book. Instead, make copies of the strategy worksheets before you get started. This way you will always have a blank template from which to work.

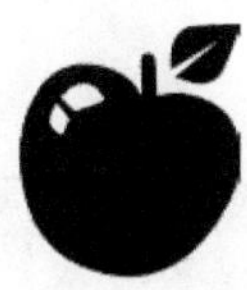

BREAKFAST

Item you eat now	Problem with it	New Solution	Benefits	New Recipe Source

LUNCH

Item you eat now	Problem with it	New Solution	Benefits	New Recipe Source

DINNER

Item you eat now	Problem with it	New Solution	Benefits	New Recipe Source

SNACKS & DESSERTS

Item you eat now	Problem with it	New Solution	Benefits	New Recipe Source

OTHER

Item you eat now	Problem with it	New Solution	Benefits	New Recipe Source

The Magic 8 Authorized Fast Food List

1 Buy already cut up butternut squash or sweet potatoes and roast them at 400-425 degrees for about 40 minutes. Spray pan and top of vegetables with non-stick cooking spray. Season vegetables as desired. You can even sprinkle pumpkin pie spice on the squash or sweet potatoes. At one of my local grocery stores, I can buy sweet potatoes already cut into sticks for fries.

2 Frozen "steam in bag" vegetables, brown rice, and wild rice and veggie mixes (no sauce or other additives).

3 Prepared fresh vegetables. Bagged and cleaned broccoli and cauliflower. Spray pan and top of veggies with non-stick cooking spray, a little salt and pepper and garlic powder – if desired – and cook at 425 degrees until they are cooked to your liking.

4 Tempeh. Warm up already seasoned tempeh or roast tofu at the same time as veggies and rice and you've got an instant meal!

5 Broccoli Slaw. Craving spaghetti and marinara sauce? Steam (in microwave is super easy) a package of broccoli slaw, add sauce, and you are done! I dare you to miss the noodles!

6 Ancient Harvest brand quinoa polenta. Slice in rounds, warm in 350 degree oven. Spray non-stick cooking spray on pan and on top of polenta rounds, warm until a bit toasty on the outside – but not dried out. You can also do this in a pan on the cooktop. Top with tomato sauce and sautéed vegetables.

7 Black bean dip (courtesy of Physicians Committee for Responsible Medicine). This dip provides an instant welcome for your guests or license to munch in front of the television.

1 can of black beans, rinsed and drained in a colander

1 small jar of salsa – whatever type you like – hot, mild, mango, etc…

Mix! An immersion blender is great for this. You can even serve it in the bowl you used to mix. Love a one dish – no pot or multiple bowls to clean – recipe!

Serve surrounded with crudités for dipping, such as baby carrots, celery sticks, mushrooms, squash and zucchini spears.

8 Eden brand organic canned rice and beans or chili. Throw one of those in your bag on your way out the door to work, and you are all set. The can is bpa-free and the food is low in sodium.

Tool #9: Healthy family activities

At the park: Go down that slide with your kids! Use the swings!

- Bring your family to local farm days for kids. There are also farm mobs and gleaning groups. Sometimes a farm needs help picking the produce. Other times they offer opportunities to pick crops for soup kitchens. All are great opportunities to connect your family to the efforts that go into bringing food to the table and the value of real food from the ground.

- Establish somewhere you go as a family every week, whether that is a free, fun park, a bounce gym, or bagels on Sunday morning. I remember going to the Hollywood Diner with my dad and my sister once a week after Hebrew school. I think they had a kid's special that night. I don't remember any main meals, any choices, any likes, dislikes, eating it, nothing. I only remember that we would always get to choose a salad dressing. My sister got ranch and I got creamy garlic. It was so good. I can smell the earthy scent of the lettuce and feel the crunch of the salad now. I am also impressed with my 6th grade self that I already liked garlic!

- Pack a picnic dinner for the pool on long summer days.

- Volunteer at a soup kitchen or food bank.

- For younger children: let them pick an animal and everyone else has to imitate it in a different way. For instance, one child orders everyone to walk like a monkey (leading the way by example of course) and the other creates a ribbiting frog race.

Tool #10: Create a YES environment

Just like grown-ups, kids need to be in a YES environment. You want to say yes instead of no. Just as you child-proof your house, or at least a play room, so that you aren't constantly telling your kids not to touch this or move that, a yes environment also applies to food.

Your children will be offered and given junk food everywhere they go. The reward from the teacher at the end of my daughter's ballet class? Lollipops made of food coloring and high fructose corn syrup.

They don't need those options in the house. In the house they need real food. I know there is a big argument out there that NOT giving your children junk food just makes them want it more outside of the house. I get that to a certain extent. However, if you have a relaxed *attitude*, that can help. If you are focusing on the number of choices in the house, rather than the number of restrictions, they will focus on that too. If you don't say a word if they go out for pizza with their friends or have a class party with cupcakes, they won't be focused on what they can't have.

In the meantime, you are setting your children up for liking healthy food for the rest of their lives. Tastes are formed in childhood. They can also change throughout life. However, your goal is to allow them to taste and love healthy, real food (not just sugar and salt that melts on the tongue) from the start. The best way to do that is to create a healthy home environment.

A yes environment is one in which your children can eat as much as they want of whatever is in the house. Children don't naturally over-eat. However, when they eat foods that are engineered in a laboratory to be addictive, their bodies and brains don't register that they are full. They aren't. Our bodies don't process fake food as real food. Pretty soon they're teenagers and then adults who no longer know what it feels like to feel truly hungry or comfortably full.

Finally, give yourself credit for where you are now.

If you are worried about how to start a conversation with your family around new foods, go around the table naming what you already like. You already eat plants. If your goal for health is to increase the number of plant based foods you eat, figure out how to expand on what you already like and what new foods you might want to try.

6

MEAL MAKEOVERS & RECIPES

The Healthy Family, Healthy You Cookbook

For over 100 additional recipes, buy *The Healthy Family, Healthy You Cookbook* on www.Amazon.com or www.HealthyFamilyHealthyYou.com. Have healthy choices at your fingertips, whether you are making a quick breakfast or hosting a holiday dinner.

Some notes before you start cooking...

If you are allergic to nuts, all or only some of them, please substitute as needed. For instance, my recipes generally call for almond milk because that is my non-dairy milk of choice. If you can only have – or simply prefer - rice, soy or something else, go ahead and use what works for you. In addition, if a recipe calls for walnuts or peanuts and you are allergic, substitute another nut, or leave them out, or just choose another recipe. There is something here for everyone.

Organic is always best. Of course it is more expensive than so-called "conventional" produce, so my hope is that the nutrients from eating lots of fruits and vegetables will make up for any harm from the pesticides. You can also look at the investment in the organic produce to be paying the farmer, rather than the doctor. A good in-between would be to buy organic for the "Dirty Dozen." Those are the 12 fruits and vegetables that are most contaminated with pesticides.

Here is the **Dirty Dozen** list from the Environmental Working Group:
Apples, Peaches, Nectarines, Strawberries, Grapes, Celery, Spinach, Sweet Bell Peppers, Cucumbers, Cherry Tomatoes, and Snap Peas (Imported). In addition, they have recently added Hot Peppers and Kale/Collard Greens.

The good news is that there are also fruits and vegetables that have low pesticide levels, even if they are not organic. The Environmental Working Group came up with a cute name for this type of produce: The Clean Fifteen. Of course you can always choose to support the health and safety of both farmers and the land by buying all organic fruits and vegetables.

The Clean Fifteen
Avocados, Sweet Corn, Pineapples, Cabbage, Sweet Peas (Frozen), Onions, Asparagus, Mangos, Papayas, Kiwi, Eggplant, Grapefruit, Cantaloupe, Cauliflower, and Sweet Potatoes.

I suggest you peel your produce if it is not organic. That's what I do with smoothies. For soups that use produce with peels, use organic produce or peel it. You don't want to make pesticide soup!

Specialty items: Many of the specialty items can be found either at your local health food store or online at Vitacost.com or on Amazon. My advice is to restock your pantry basics one at a time. You don't need to buy 15 new items each week, unless you want to and can afford to!

Meal Makeovers

Key:
In italics: A typical day on the Standard American Diet (SAD)
See all healthy recipes below
In bold: Your new Healthy Family, Healthy You day

BREAKFAST
SAD: Store-bought muffin
Healthy: Chocolate Chip Banana Muffins

SNACK
SAD: Pudding cup
Healthy: Chia Pudding

LUNCH
SAD: Chinese Take-out
Healthy: Chinese Orange No-Chicken Salad

AFTERNOON PICK-ME-UP
SAD: Frappuccino
Healthy: Healthy Homemade Nutella Frappuccino

DINNER
SAD: Lasagna made with ground beef and 3 types of cheese (ricotta, mozzarella, and parmesan)
Healthy: Non-Dairy, Gluten-Free Lasagna

DESSERT
SAD: Traditional fruit crumble made with butter and flour
Healthy: Pear Crumble

I've provided pictures and links to many of the ingredients in this book and the companion cookbook, on my website. Go to www.healthyfamilyhealthyyou.com/pantrylist.

Chocolate Banana Mini-Muffins

Makes 24 mini muffins

You won't find a healthier or easier recipe than this! These make a great grab and go breakfast, snack, or even a treat at lunch.

This is a variation of my recipe (on my website and in the cookbook) for granola bars/cookies.

3 large bananas
3/4 cup quick oats
1/4 cup ground walnuts (can substitute another ground nut or leave out entirely for allergy issues)
1/4 cup flax meal
Dash of real vanilla
Dash of cinnamon
1/8 cup mini chocolate chips

Heat oven to 350 degrees. Mash bananas with a fork in a mixing bowl. Add oats, walnuts and flax meal, cinnamon and vanilla. Mix well. Add chocolate chips and mix again.

Put mini cupcake liners into your mini cupcake pan and then spray the liners with non-stick spray. Place approximately 1 Tablespoon of batter in each muffin liner. This recipe makes EXACTLY 24 mini muffins-the same number as in my mini muffin tin.

Bake in center of oven for 15 minutes. They won't look quite done, but they are. Let cool for a few minutes so no little kiddies (or adults) burn their tongues on the hot (yummy!) chocolate chips. Refrigerate after cooling.

Tip: You can mix in different nuts (whole or ground) and dried fruit, depending on your preferences. However, I will tell you that I tried coconut flakes and their flavor really got lost.

Ch-Ch-Ch-Chia... Pudding!

Serves 1-2

Watching those Chia Head commercials growing up, did you ever imagine it would become the next Super Food? Did you know what a Super Food or Kale was? Chances are, you did not. I know I did not and my parents were always into healthy food.

Per your request, here is the basic recipe (and some fun options) for the chia pudding I tricked my kids into eating. It's not really a trick…it's just reverse psychology. I eat it. It is MY food. Then they want it.

Oh and in case you did not know, I wanted to trick my kids into eating it because it is full of healthy plant protein, antioxidants and omega fats.

Basic Recipe:
1/4 cup chia seeds
2/3 cup water (You can also substitute chocolate or vanilla almond or other non-dairy milk. Canned coconut milk will make it especially rich.)
1 Tablespoon maple syrup or agave nectar

Optional additions: sliced fruit, nuts, toasted unsweetened coconut, dash of cinnamon (Add these right before serving)

2 great versions that I love:
Chocolate Banana: Use unsweetened chocolate almond milk, agave nectar and bananas.
Vanilla Berry: Use unsweetened vanilla almond milk, maple syrup, blueberries and strawberries.

Mix the chia seeds with the water (or milk substitute) and sweetener; cover and place the bowl in the fridge to firm up. The minimum for this is 10 minutes, but the longer you leave it in, the firmer it will become. For breakfast, it is easiest to make this the night before. Then, in the morning, just pull it out, mix and add any optional ingredients of your choice. If making it as a dessert, put the pudding together and refrigerate before you start making the meal.

Tasha's Tip: You will want to mix it well when you take it out of the fridge. In addition, if you are leaving it in for longer than the 10 minutes, feel free to give it a mix once or twice if you think of it.

Chinese Orange No-Chicken Salad

Serves 4

Even if you are sure your kids will never like tofu, try this recipe. They will!

Orange Tofu

1 pound package extra firm tofu, pressed*
3 TB orange marmalade (please find one without high fructose corn syrup and with pieces of orange peel still inside).

Heat oven to 425 degrees. Press tofu (see directions below). Dice tofu into 1 inch cubes. Mix gently with the orange marmalade, being careful not to mush the tofu. Place parchment paper on a large cookie sheet. Spray with non-stick spray. Lay the cubes out on the parchment paper, preferably not touching so that they will be able to roast, rather than steam. Spray the top of the tofu with non-stick spray or olive oil. Cook at 425 degrees until slightly browned and hardened to consistency of chicken breast, about 20 minutes. Allow to cool.

Salad

2 romaine hearts, chopped
1 red pepper, diced
1 cup baby carrots, each carrot cut in thirds.
1 15 oz can or jar mandarin oranges, drained (2 TB liquid reserved for dressing)
1 cup toasted peanuts
1 cup egg-free crunchy Chinese noodles

Wash and dry the romaine. Tear or cut it into bite sized pieces. Add romaine to a large bowl. Top with rest of the salad ingredients (except garnish) and the no-chicken orange tofu.

Dressing
¼ cup brown rice vinegar
2 Tablespoons maple syrup
2 Tablespoons safflower oil
4 Tablespoons orange marmalade
2 Tablespoons juice from can or jar of mandarin oranges

Combine all ingredients in a glass jar and shake until emulsified.

Toss the salad with the dressing. Garnish and serve.

*To press tofu: Place a stack of 8 paper towels onto a large plate. Open the tofu container and drain the liquid. Place the entire block of tofu on top of the paper towels. Place another layer of 8 paper towels on top of the tofu. Take a heavy dish (such as a ceramic baking dish) and place it on top of the tofu. Make sure everything is balanced and it won't crash down onto or off your counter! Leave for at least 30 minutes. If you want, you can also do this in the morning and then leave the whole contraption in the fridge for the day while you are out. When you come home, the tofu will ready to go.

Nutella Frappuccino

Serves 2-4

After you see the name of this recipe, you will be running to get the ingredients to make it!

2 cups chocolate non-dairy milk
4 teaspoons instant coffee granules or powder (use decaf for the kids)
2 Tablespoons hazelnut soy or coconut milk vegan creamer
(If using unsweetened non-dairy milk, add 1 Tablespoon agave nectar.)
2 frozen bananas*
2 cups ice

Warm chocolate plant based milk for 45 seconds in the microwave. Pour into blender. Dissolve instant coffee granules into the milk. Add the rest of the ingredients (except ice) and blend. Add ice and blend again.

***How to freeze bananas:** Even if you don't have time or patience to make banana bread, you will never have an excuse for wasting too-ripe bananas again! For the best tasting smoothie, you will want to freeze your bananas. To do this, you should start with a ripe banana. Peel the banana (this is critical) and then you can break it in half or thirds (smaller pieces will make blending easier). If you have more patience than I do and want to make sure your bananas never have a hint of freezer burn, you can wrap each banana in plastic wrap before placing it in a freezer bag. If you have glass containers that freeze and prefer that to plastic, you can use those too; but then you should definitely wrap the bananas in plastic wrap, or they will become freezer burned.

Best Ever Lasagna (Gluten-free!)

Serves 6-8

This lasagna has become such a hit with my friends that they request it when they come for meals. They don't tell their kids about the tofu or spinach until they are gobbling it up…and they always gobble it up!

1 16-ounce bag of chopped, frozen spinach
1 cup frozen, chopped onion
1 12 or 14-ounce box frozen butternut squash puree (or bpa-free can)
1 1 lb package organic silken tofu
1 32-ounce jar pasta sauce (Pick any flavor you like. I often use garlic or mushroom)
1/2-1 teaspoon each garlic powder, dried thyme and Italian seasoning
1 package brown rice lasagna noodles (like Tinkyada, 10 ounce)
1 24-ounce jar roasted red peppers (about 3 whole peppers)
1/8 cup gluten-free panko bread crumbs (if gluten-free isn't necessary for you, use whole wheat)
1/8 cup nutritional yeast

Heat oven to 350 degrees. Spray bottom of 13" x 9" lasagna pan with non-stick cooking spray.

Place frozen spinach, onion and squash into a large glass bowl and defrost in the microwave (I use the "vegetable" setting).

Place tofu into bowl with defrosted vegetables. Add thyme, garlic powder and Italian seasoning and mix thoroughly.

Place one layer of noodles in pan, followed by half of the vegetable and tofu mix. Cover with 1/3 of the bottle of marinara sauce. Spread it thinly and evenly.

Place another layer of noodles in the pan. Cover with the rest of the vegetable tofu mix and another third of the marinara sauce.

Place your final layer of noodles in the pan. Cover with the rest of the marinara sauce and then the roasted red peppers (cut open and flatten if still whole).

Mix the Panko bread crumbs and nutritional yeast together in a small bowl. Sprinkle evenly over the top of the red peppers.

Cook for 1 hour, uncovered, at 350 degrees.

Pear Crumble

Serves 4-6

I bought pears the other day that tasted like mealy cardboard. I cooked them into a crisp, and the pears tasted like candy.

2 large or 4 small very ripe pears
½ cup oats
¼ cup coconut sugar (or light brown sugar or skip it all together…)
1 teaspoon vanilla
½ teaspoon cinnamon
¼ cup apple sauce

Heat oven to 350 degrees. Spray 8" x 8" ceramic baking dish with non-stick spray. Dice pears, leaving skin on. Place into baking dish. Mix oats, sugar, vanilla and cinnamon in a small bowl. Add apple sauce and mix well. Top the pears with the oat and apple sauce mixture, spreading it evenly over the top of the dish.

Bake uncovered at 350 degrees for about an hour.

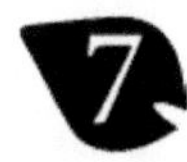

RESOURCES

Resource Guide

The following are resources that have proven helpful to me, day in and day out, as I have transformed my own diet and that of my family. I hope that you will discover additional resources on your own. There are always more out there. However, you don't want to read a 20 page list and neither would I. In the meantime, the items on this list will provide you with a solid foundation of knowledge, support and encouragement, with which to start your own journey.

Every day I have to restrain myself from buying another vegan cookbook. There are so many good ones out there! I own so many, but I use them all. I never have a shortage of meal ideas. Check out this list so you feel that way too!

When you cook from a low fat vegan/plant based cookbook, you don't have to count calories or think about portions and food groups. You will naturally eat a varied diet and stop eating when you are full.

In the lists below you might notice a number of related, repeated items. No, I did not cut and paste one too many times! For instance, *Forks over Knives* started as a movie, became a book and spawned a cookbook. That's just one example of several related sets of books/movies/cookbooks in the whole foods, plant based (WFPB) world. In addition, a number of the non-cookbook books also contain recipes.

Trust me; they're all worth checking out!

Websites

Whole Foods Plant Based Info www.wfpb411.com

Katie Oliver adopted a whole foods, plant based diet in January of 2013. Since then she has lost weight and feels great. She started her blog to help others learn how to become what she calls a "healthy vegan." She says, "The main difference is that WFPB means you follow the rules of a vegan regarding animals, but you eat "Whole" foods... UNPROCESSED foods like fruits, vegetables, beans, nuts, whole grains, etc." In several sections of the website, she shows how some processed foods appear healthy, but are not actually made of (only) whole foods. She then provides an alternative home-made recipe. Oliver provides her recipes, and those of her favorite vegan bloggers. You will find many resources and recipes here.

Veg News Magazine www.vegnews.com

I like Veg News magazine more than its main competitor, Vegetarian Times, because it contains healthier recipes, without any animal products. Vegetarian Times is a very useful magazine if you want to use eggs and dairy, but not chicken or beef, in most of your recipes. I don't, so I stick to Veg News. I even enjoy the advertisements because it is a great way to learn about new products that might be helpful for my healthy and vegan lifestyle.

Averie Cooks www.averiecooks.com

With the tag line, "Recipes for Sweet Teeth," this may seem like a strange recommendation from me. Although most of her recipes are of the egg, butter and flour filled variety, there are a number of vegan, and even somewhat healthy recipes. The caramels (made from pine nuts) and chocolate chip cookie dough (made from cashews) alone are worth a trip to the website. Click on Browse Recipes and then Recipe Index. There you will find categories such as vegan, vegetarian and gluten-free. Apparently, Averie Sunshine does not live on sweets alone, evidenced by her slim physique (due to her self-proclaimed love of yoga and running, I presume) and healthy real food recipes, such as smoothies, The Green Powerhouse Salad and Do-It-Yourself Guacamole Bar. Last 4th of July I made her Caramelized Onion and Portobello Mushroom Sliders with Fry Sauce. All the carnivores wanted some!

Physician's Committee for Responsible Medicine www.pcrm.org

As you know by now, I am a big fan of PCRM. Their website contains numerous resources for physicians, consumers and policy makers, including scientific research, legislative information and their free Vegetarian Starter Kit, with a Kickstart program running each month. This program is available in 4 languages.

NutritionMD www.nutritionmd.org

This website is associated with PCRM, and provides information for physicians, consumers, those who are already vegetarian but looking to fine tune the healthfulness of their diet, and those with concerns about specific health issues. When I am looking for a recipe, especially when I have a specific ingredient in mind, this is one of the first places I look. In addition, they now have a FREE meal planner that will generate nutrition information and a shopping list.

Dr. Joel Fuhrman www.drfuhrman.com

A prolific author and physician, Dr. Fuhrman's website provides several membership levels with a range of benefits; a personal nutrition-counseling program; scientific information about the relationship between food and a number of different diseases; and recipes and products to support a healthy, plant based lifestyle. He sells his own line of vitamins, salad dressings, flavored vinegars, soups and even healthful ketchup.

Choosing Raw www.choosingraw.com

Choosing Raw is Amy Hamshaw's blog and the name of her book. She is a certified clinical nutritionist who offers nutritional counseling and recipes from dips and sauces to small plates and smoothies. If you need a recipe idea for any meal, you will find it here. Her thoughtful blog posts address ethical and physical reasons for eating raw and vegan and also the range of emotional issues surrounding food and life balance, making her website more than just a recipe resource. She also specifically addresses many facets of eating disorders, including her own journey and recovery.

Fat Free Vegan www.fatfreevegan.com

So many times when I am looking for a specific recipe, I may find it vegan, but that doesn't mean it is not full of fat, flour and sugar. When I go to Fat Free Vegan, I know what I am going to find. Susan Voisin's recipes are made with whole foods and without added oil. Some recipes do include avocados, nuts or coconut, all sources of healthy and essential fats. However, as Voisin writes on her website, "Oil-Free Vegan" just did not sound like such a great website name and Fat Free Vegan was born. The website contains over 1400 recipes developed by Voisin and her readers.

Chocolate Covered Katie www.chocolatecoveredkatie.com

Name your favorite treat. Anything. Chances are, you will find a better version on this healthy dessert blog (with main meal ideas too). Katie Higgins has also written a *Chocolate Covered Katie* cookbook with over 80 healthy dessert recipes. Who wants one minute chocolate cake or healthy imitations of popular candy cars? I'm in! She also provides healthy breakfast recipes, including grab and go options. She started writing new versions of her favorite treats to tame her own sugar habit. Run, don't walk, to this website!

Food Babe www.foodbabe.com

Food Babe is such an effective investigator and advocate for consumers that the big food corporations and lobbies are doing everything they can to destroy her. Food Babe (real name: Vani Hari) has her own story of a health transformation through eating well. However, she did not stop at changing her own diet and educating others to do the same. She investigates questionable ingredients and practices in some of the biggest restaurants and food manufacturers. She and the "food babe army," as she calls her followers, have used their pens, computers and dollars to bring about big changes at big food companies. She also offers recipes and food guides for individuals. Also, fyi, she is not a vegan. She does consume (and include in her recipes) organic eggs and dairy. This could be a good resource for those not interested in going totally vegan.

Cookbooks

The Food Babe Way: Break Free from the Hidden Toxins in Your Food and Lose Weight, Look Years Younger, and Get Healthy in Just 21 Days!
By Vani Hari (February 10, 2015)
This is the new book by the aforementioned blogger and food industry investigator. This book will help you understand the food industry, the dangers of processed foods, and give you a 21 day plan to detoxify and feel great.

Chocolate-Covered Katie: Over 80 Delicious Recipes That Are Secretly Good for You
by Katie Higgins (January 6, 2015)
This is the new book from the aforementioned blogger, a gorgeous and thin young woman who eats chocolate every day!

Choosing Raw: Making Raw Foods Part of the Way You Eat
by Amy Hamshaw (July 1, 2014)
This is the book from Amy Hamshaw of the Choosing Raw website, recommended above. She is a certified clinical nutritionist and pre-med, post-bachelor's degree. She suggests that everyone can benefit from adding more raw food to their diets, but chooses to eat (and provide recipes for) both raw and cooked (always vegan) foods. The book includes 125 recipes and 21 days of plant based meal plans.

Mayim's Vegan Table: More than 100 Great-Tasting and Healthy Recipes from My Family to Yours
by Mayim Bialik (Feb 11, 2014)
Mayim's recipes are fairly easy and straight-forward, in addition to veganizing many children's typical favorite foods. It is a valuable and practical starter cookbook for families. However, many of her recipes are filled with sugar, flour, vegan margarine and fake meats and cheeses. I am personally moving away from that and recommending

that others do the same. Nevertheless, I do recommend this book, especially for beginning families.

Better Than Vegan: 101 Favorite Low-Fat, Plant-Based Recipes That Helped Me Lose Over 200 Pounds

by Del Sroufe (Dec 3, 2013)

If there is ever any one to remind us that flour and sugar are vegan and that vegan doesn't necessarily equally healthy, it is Sroufe, formerly a 400 plus pound vegan pastry chef who owned his own bakery. Sroufe faced his food addiction and emerged a new type of chef; a fit one who provides many recipes for practical basics (such as cream sauce made from cauliflower and and sweetener syrup made from dates), along with meal recipes.

Forks Over Knives - The Cookbook: Over 300 Recipes for Plant based Eating All Through the Year

by Del Sroufe, Julieanna Hever MS RD CPT, Isa Chandra Moskowitz and Darshana Thacker (Aug 14, 2012)

If you buy one cookbook, perhaps it should be this one. I don't think there is any type of food you won't find in this dense book, from cornbread to chocolate cake. It is kind of like an encyclopedia and bible in one!

The China Study Cookbook: Over 120 Whole Food, Plant-Based Recipes

by LeAnne Campbell, Steven Campbell Disla and T. Colin Campbell (May 7, 2013)

This is the cookbook based on the advice in T. Colin Campbell's book, *The China Study.*

Fresh from the Vegan Slow Cooker: 200 Ultra-Convenient, Super-Tasty, Completely Animal-Free Recipes
by Robin Robertson (Sept 25, 2012)
From Shepherd's pie to "Artisanal sweet and spice wiener balls," Robertson covers many family favorites, using handy and familiar ingredients. We all forget that the slow cooker can really help us. I use this book to remind myself!

Vegan with a Vengeance: Over 150 Delicious, Cheap, Animal-Free Recipes That Rock
by Isa Chandra Moskowitz (Oct 28, 2005)
This was Moskowitz's first cookbook and you can feel her youth and spunky personality come through the pages. You will also love the easy, down to earth (yet inspired) recipes, whether you are cooking brunch for you and your significant other, or throwing a dinner party for 25.

Appetite for Reduction: 125 Fast and Filling Low-Fat Vegan Recipes
by Isa Chandra Moskowitz and Matthew Ruscigno (Dec 7, 2010)
The recipes in this book contain significantly less sugar and flour than *Vegan with a Vengeance.* They are surprisingly satisfying, as the title implies, and a great go-to book when you want to watch your fat and calories, without sacrificing flavor and creativity. But don't stop here. Moskowitz's other cookbooks are also slam-dunks. I trust you will have as hard of a time as I did choosing which ones to purchase.

Wild About Greens: 125 Delectable Vegan Recipes for Kale, Collards, Arugula, Bok Choy, and other Leafy Veggies Everyone Loves
by Nava Atlas (Jun 5, 2012)
We all go to the store, feeling virtuous, and buy up bunches of bright and exotic greens. Then we get home and have no idea what to do

with them. Between the techniques and recipes Atlas provides, you will never have this problem again. If you need to eat your greens, you will find a way inside this book. Just like Moskowitz, above, you will have a hard time choosing which of her numerous cookbooks to buy. This woman just never runs out of recipes or ideas!

Vegan Holiday Kitchen: More than 200 Delicious, Festive Recipes for Special Occasions
by Nava Atlas and Susan Voisin (Nov 1, 2011)
I love this book and use it all year round. It is for everyone. From Christian to Jewish to American holidays and occasions, she has you covered. You will find both recipes and complete menus for events ranging from the Fourth of July, to Easter, along with menus for both Sephardic and Ashkenazi Passover Seders. She doesn't miss anything!

The Get Healthy, Go Vegan Cookbook: 125 Easy and Delicious Recipes to Jump-Start Weight Loss and Help You Feel Great.
by Neal Barnard and Robyn Webb (Jun 8, 2010)
These simple recipes are a great place to start when looking for healthy and plant based alternatives to your usual fare. The encouraging tone, straight-forward nutrition information, shopping lists and convenience foods, make this book a basic starter for anyone looking to shift their diet.

Cooking with Trader Joe's Cookbook: Skinny Dish!
by Jennifer K. Reilly and Heather World (Oct 15, 2011)
I met Jennifer K. Reilly at a women's event for my synagogue. I was tickled to later figure out that she used to work at PCRM and wrote a cookbook with Dr. Neil Barnard! She is a registered dietician and a busy mom with a contagious zest for life and healthy eating. She doesn't have time to make it complicated and she knows most of us

don't either. The book contains practical tips for a skinny lifestyle, along with recipes for healthy and vegan versions of your favorite foods, like nachos, chicken salad and mozzarella sticks. Whether you are single or have a big family, you need her ideas for easy, healthy versions of football game appetizers and 15 minute dinners. Everything, including a detox plan, is in here!

Eat to Live Cookbook: 200 Delicious Nutrient-Rich Recipes for Fast and Sustained Weight Loss, Reversing Disease, and Lifelong Health
by Joel Fuhrman (Oct 8, 2013)
This is the cookbook that expands on Dr. Fuhrman's original, foundational book, *Eat to Live.* It contains the quick and dirty version of his previous nutritional advice, along with recipes that include everything you might expect, plus blended salads, non vegan foods and his own fast food list.

Gluten-Free Recipes for the Conscious Cook: A Seasonal, Vegetarian Cookbook (The New Harbinger Whole-Body Healing Series)
by Leslie Cerier and Kathie Swift MS RD (July 1, 2010)
I met Cerier at the Hazon Food Conference several years ago. Anyone who has celiac disease or is serious about going gluten-free should check out this book. It is full of both basic and creative recipes with many new grains that may be unfamiliar to you.

The Beauty Detox Power: Nourish Your Mind and Body for Weight Loss and Discover True Joy Paperback
by Kimberly Snyder (March 31, 2015)
Snyder is a nutritionist to the stars and an avid yogi. This new book of hers is the third in her Beauty Detox series. She combines recipes designed to promote different chakras and stories of clients she's

helped over the years, with a focus on what can stop us from becoming healthier.

The Beauty Detox Foods: Discover the Top 50 Beauty Foods That Will Transform Your Body and Reveal a More Beautiful You
by Kimberly Snyder (March 26, 2013)
There are recipes from this book that I return to time and time again (such as raw vegan tacos made from ground walnuts and spices) and others I just don't have it in me to try (like recipes that require me to ferment my own food). Once you see how healthy she looks, you will become a follower. Many recipes do require ingredients that may be new to you, but I encourage you to buy those kelp granules and get started! I recently had the pleasure of visiting her Glow Bio raw food and juice bar in Los Angeles and I kind of wanted to move in!

Non-fiction Books

Whole: Rethinking the Science of Nutrition
by T. Colin Campbell and Howard Jacobson (May 7, 2013)

Forks Over Knives: The Plant Based Way to Health
by Gene Stone, T. Colin Campbell and Caldwell B. Esselstyn (June 28, 2011)

The China Study: The Most Comprehensive Study of Nutrition Ever Conducted and the Startling Implications for Diet, Weight Loss, and Long-term Health
by T. Colin Campbell, Thomas M. Campbell II (May 11, 2006)

The Engine 2 Diet: The Texas Firefighter's 28-Day Save-Your-Life Plan that Lowers Cholesterol and Burns Away the Pounds
by Rip Esselstyn (2009)

The End of Dieting: How to Live for Life
by Joel Fuhrman (March 25, 2014)

Eat For Health
by Joel Fuhrman (Sep 1, 2012)

Disease-Proof Your Child: Feeding Kids Right
by Joel Fuhrman (Sep 5, 2006)

Eat to Live: The Revolutionary Formula for Fast and Sustained Weight Loss
by Joel Fuhrman and Mehmet Oz (Jan 5, 2005)

Your Food Is Fooling You: How Your Brain Is Hijacked by Sugar, Fat, and Salt
by David A. Kessler (Dec 24, 2012)

The End of Overeating: Taking Control of the Insatiable American Appetite
by David A. Kessler (Sep 14, 2010)

Fat Chance: Beating the Odds Against Sugar, Processed Food, Obesity, and Disease
by Robert H. Lustig (Dec 27, 2012)

Salt Sugar Fat: How the Food Giants Hooked Us
by Michael Moss (Feb 26, 2013)

No More Dirty Looks: The Truth about Your Beauty Products--and the Ultimate Guide to Safe and Clean Cosmetics
by Siobhan O'Connor and Alexandra Spunt (July 13, 2010)

Other specialty books

Dr. Neal Barnard's Program for Reversing Diabetes: The Scientifically Proven System for Reversing Diabetes without Drugs.
by Neal D. Barnard (Apr 1, 2008)

The End of Diabetes: The Eat to Live Plan to Prevent and Reverse Diabetes
by Joel Fuhrman (Dec 26, 2012)

Power Foods for the Brain: An Effective 3-Step Plan to Protect Your Mind and Strengthen Your Memory
by Neal Barnard (Feb 19, 2013)

Breaking the Food Seduction: The Hidden Reasons Behind Food Cravings---And 7 Steps to End Them Naturally
by Neal D. Barnard and Joanne Stepaniak (Sep 23, 2004)

Foods That Fight Pain: Proven Dietary Solutions for Maximum Pain Relief Without Drugs
by Neal D. Barnard (2008)

The Cancer Survivor's Guide: Foods That Help You Fight Back
by Neal Barnard and Jennifer K. Reilly (Jan 15, 2009)

Foods That Cause You to Lose Weight: The Negative Calorie Effect
by Neal Barnard (Apr 26, 2011)

Prevent and Reverse Heart Disease: The Revolutionary, Scientifically Proven, Nutrition-Based Cure
by Caldwell B. Esselstyn, Jr. (Jan 31, 2008)

Movies

Food, Inc., starring Eric Schlosser (2008)
Food Matters, starring Andrew W. Saul, Charlotte Gerson, Dr. Dan Rogers, et al. (2009)

Vegucated, starring T. Colin Campbell, Brian Flegel, Joel Fuhrman, et al. (2010)

Planeat, starring T. Colin Campbell, Caldwell Esselstyn, Jr. Shelley Lee Davies (Director), Or Shlomi (Director) (2010)

Fat, Sick & Nearly Dead, starring Joe Cross (2010)

Forks Over Knives, starring T. Colin Campbell, Caldwell B. Esselstyn, Jr., et al. (2011)

Milk?, starring Sebastian Howard (Director), Neal Barnard (2012)

Fat, Sick & Nearly Dead 2, starring Joe Cross (2014)

Food

For a pantry list, along with pictures and links to ingredients that might be new to you, go to www.healthyfamilyhealthyyou.com/pantrylist.

Pasta

Tinkyada brown rice pasta
Tofu shiratake noodles
Bean spaghetti (aduki, black, mung bean and soy)
Barilla pasta with vegetables already cooked in (This is not made with whole grain flour. However, every bit of fruits and veggies helps and so does extra color, texture and flavor)
Broccoli slaw (as a substitute for pasta)

Thickeners

Organic corn starch
Tapiocas
Agar agar
Guar gum

Fruit

Brother's all natural dehydrated fruit crisps
Rehydrate for an add-in at the last minute when you don't have fresh fruit available or time to deal with it. I throw it in my oatmeal Tupperware as I'm running out the door. By the time I get to the office, it is all soft and yummy. Super concentrated sweetness. Banana and strawberry in oatmeal. Yum! Or you can reconstitute it in hot water and use for muffins.
Little Duck's tiny fruits

Beans

Low-sodium cans of pinto, black, great northern, cannellini, black eyed peas, kidney beans. Several brands, such as Eden, make organic beans in a BPA-free can.

Desserts

Sprinkles without food coloring and natural versions of food coloring can be found in your local health food store. They use natural food sources to make a rainbow of different cake and cookie decorations.
Dandies vegan marshmallows (Chicago Vegan Foods)
Ricemellow is the vegan version of marshmallow fluff

Grains

Barley, black rice, brown rice, quinoa, oatmeal (steel cut, old fashioned and oat groats), buckwheat groats

Fast food

Eden Foods cans of rice and beans or chili.
Eden foods cans don't contain BPA, a hormone disruptor, like almost every other can on the market.
Low-sodium veggie broth
Ancient Harvest quinoa polenta
Keep cans of baby beets or matchstick beets on hand
(See the *Healthy Family, Healthy You* cookbook for an easy, yet impressive, last-second beet salad)

Fats

Coconut, sesame, and extra virgin olive oils
Non-hydrogenated vegan margarine

Frozen

Fruit, veggies, brown rice, wild rice with veggies

Trader Joe's is a great store for affordable organic frozen veggies, rice and fruit. Look for their green and yellow bean mix with carrots. It looks really nice, not like it was frozen, and the carrots are very sweet. This mix is great for both kids and company.

Also, try bulk clubs for affordable frozen fruits and veggies.

Flours

Coconut, oat, buckwheat, spelt, whole wheat pastry, white whole wheat, whole grain corn meal, chickpea and brown rice

Milk

Almond, rice, hemp, soy, cashew and coconut milks

Be sure to look for unsweetened (and chocolate!) options.

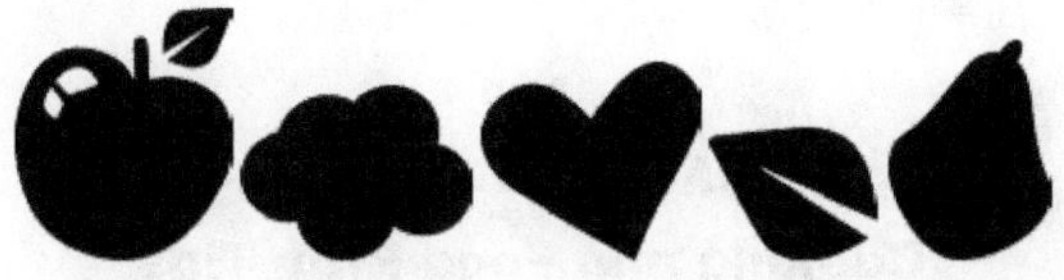

TASHA'S TIPS AND TRICKS!

50! Tasha's Tips and Tricks

What to eat
What NOT to Eat
Cooking and Food Prep Tips
Tricks are for Kids!
Kitchen Equipment
Strategies for Clarity

What TO Eat

Keep **eating plants**! You already eat plants. Think of the fruits, vegetables and legumes you already like. Now, eat more of them!

Try new plants! Most people who switch to a plant based diet actually think they eat a larger variety of foods, rather than feeling limited, as they might have suspected.

Don't worry about food combining at each meal, like dieticians suggested in the old days. If you **eat a variety of fruits, vegetables, whole grains and legumes throughout the day**, you won't have to go out of your way to make a "complete protein" from two vegetarian sources.

Buy **brown rice cakes** instead of crackers. Sometimes you can even substitute them for bread. Look for the small square ones usually carried in a store's kosher section.

Coconut milk and soy creamer are both **delicious in coffee**. Most "non-dairy" creamer actually has dairy! Hint – look at the allergy info that packages are now carrying. It will say: contains: soy, dairy, wheat, eggs, etc… so you will know for sure. Sometimes it will just say it is produced on the same equipment, which is fine. Order powdered soy creamer that you can carry in your purse or pocket. www.soygo.net

Tips for buying bread: Look for bread with only a few ingredients, such as flour, salt, yeast. There are often small bakeries and chains offering this. Find one in your neighborhood. In the regular grocery store, there is usually only one brand (Bakers) that fits the bill. Small, dense breads containing almost nothing aside from rye or pumpernickel flour (good break from so much wheat!) can be found at Trader Joe's or your local health food store. Be sure to check the sodium content.

Use **sunflower butter** where peanut/nut butter isn't allowed. My kids don't even know the difference if I give them peanut butter, almond butter or sunflower butter. Just like nut butters, try to buy sunflower butter without additives. It is delicious when the only ingredient is sunflower seeds. No salt or oil or preservatives necessary! (Be sure to make sure none of your child's classmates are allergic to seeds, but an allergy to sunflower seeds is pretty rare. Also, be sure to tell your child's teacher or camp counselor that it is sunflower butter, because it looks just like peanut butter, and they might freak out that you are breaking the rules.)

Cinnamon helps regulate blood sugar. Just a teaspoon a day can help control hunger and cravings, whether or not you are at risk for diabetes.

Sweet potatoes are a great fast food! Buy small ones, wash them, put them in the microwave, hit the potato button, and you are done. Larger sweet potatoes may not be finished after the microwave cycle. Simply wrap them in a dish towel to finish cooking. They are also much easier to peel after they have been cooked and cooled. It will take five seconds with your hands. No calluses and sore back from the peeler. At one of my local chain grocery stores they sell sweet potatoes already peeled and cut into fries and chunks. I buy them occasionally (see my low down cheatin' cholent recipe in the Healthy Family, Healthy You cookbook) but always make sure to inspect them to make sure they are fresh enough.

To **replace eggs** when baking, you have several choices:

1. Chia egg: For 1 egg, combine 3 Tablespoons water and 1 Tablespoon white chia seed meal (Grind in a spice grinder yourself, or don't grind if your recipe can handle it. You can also use black chia seeds, if your recipe can handle it aesthetically!) Let it sit for 5 or 10 minutes until it is gelatinous, before using.

2. Flax meal egg: To replace 1 egg, combine 3 Tablespoons water and 1 Tablespoon ground flax meal (purchased ground and kept in the refrigerator or freshly ground). Add the water to the flax meal and mix well with a fork. Let it set for about 15 minutes, preferably in the fridge. Mix again and add to your recipe.

3. Egg replacer powder: The most common brand is Ener-G, available at any health food store, and it is mixed with water. If your recipe demands any type of rising, get it in the oven right away after making/adding the "egg."

4. Replace each egg with 1 small banana. This can work well with cake mixes.

If you are not very experienced in baking without eggs, follow a number of vegan recipes first, and then you will get a feel for which substitute might work best in other recipes that do call for eggs.

Replace oil. Use apple sauce as a 1 to 1 replacement in cake recipes. In addition, you can also use apple sauce as a replacement for oil or butter when making streusel to top fresh fruit or cakes.

Eat cocoa! Minimally-processed cocoa powder actually contains more antioxidants than blueberries! Isn't that the best news since sliced bread?! Hershey's now makes a special cocoa powder where cocoa powder is the only ingredient. However, the majority of Hershey's cocoa powder is alkali processed (also called Dutch processed) and does not contain the antioxidants you want. Even better...cacao powder, found at the health food store, is much richer in taste than commercial brands of cocoa powder and is the unprocessed version of cocoa, with three to four times as many antioxidants. Make sure it is fair trade, and you have really contributed to world peace!

Use **Tiny Fruits** (a brand found online and in health food stores) dehydrated apples and bananas as crunchy bits instead of granola or candy. Right now, many kids are obsessed with the junk food candy crunch yogurt. Instead, try coconut milk or other non-dairy yogurt with the Tiny Fruits.

Use **plant based milks**. Most are interchangeable with dairy milk in recipes. Use rice if you want the taste to be as non-existent as possible.

Salad dressing. Have a little trans fat, sugar, food coloring, MSG and preservatives with your salad? Make your own salad dressing! It is actually very easy. You don't even need added oil to make it delicious. Look online for healthy recipes, use your new vegan cookbooks or simply combine some balsamic vinegar with mustard or lemon juice and fresh herbs, like parsley and basil. Use nuts, seeds or avocado in place of oil. Done!

Popcorn. Use an old school air popper with (preferably organic, non-GMO) popcorn kernels. Spray on some olive oil and grind a little pink Himalayan sea salt and I promise it will taste like movie popcorn!

Identify a place in your area where you can get **healthy "take-out."** For instance, in my area there is a vegan, healthy soup shop called Souper Girl that will even deliver. Native Foods, a national vegan fast(ish) food chain just opened two locations in Washington, DC. Puree Juice in Bethesda carries fresh juices, smoothies and raw, vegan takeout meals. Unless you live in a rural area, you will probably find a good option. If you do live in a rural area without such places, work with a local restaurant to create a few healthy menu options. Then, take your friends! Both your friends and the restaurant owners will find out that this type of food is needed and wanted.

What NOT to Eat

You can't have your cake and eat it too: Unfortunately, a**ll soda is unhealthy**. However, naturally flavored seltzer is not. Buying a seltzer machine (such as a Soda Stream) will help the kids get into this alternative. In addition, even if you do make them cola soda with the machine (only occasionally!), it will have less sugar than soda in the store.

Artificial sweeteners don't help with weight gain or sugar cravings. In fact, they do the opposite. I promise that you can find healthier, low sugar recipes for your favorite foods, without resorting to using artificial sweeteners.

When trying to change your diet and take out animal products, don't ADD IN **fake food**. Trust me, I have done the experimenting for you – there are not any fake cheeses out there that will taste, smell or feel like real cheese. Occasionally, I do crave a "deli" sandwich, and then I'll use the fake deli. But other than occasional treats, try to stick to whole foods.

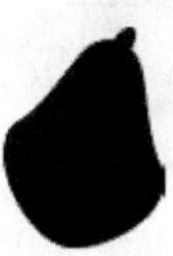

Cooking & Food Prep

If you buy fresh greens, fruit or other vegetables, always try to **freeze** them if you think you might not use them before they start to degrade. (Some, like corn, require blanching before freezing). Frozen fruit and greens, no matter how it looks or the consistency (even lettuce) can be thrown into a smoothie or soup.

If you have a Vitamix, throw in your vegetables before they go bad and **make soup**. If you don't have a Vitamix, use an immersion blender. Stay away from the usual canned soups as much as possible. There are healthy vegan soups without tons of sodium and MSG out there for the time starved. Try www.DrFuhrman.com for packs you can leave in the office or open quickly on a weeknight. Those, however, are the exception (and they are not cheap), so it is a great idea to learn to make your own.

Use s**moked paprika**, instead of lots of salt, on homemade fries or baked potatoes.

Make your own **croutons**. It is so easy, and then they won't taste like a cardboard box; you will know the sodium content isn't insane; and you will know it hasn't been sitting on the shelf for months. With spices like smoked paprika and garlic, who needs salt? I had leftover cranberry cornbread (great www.pcrm.org recipe!) so, I made croutons and put them on butternut squash-coconut milk soup (thank you Dafna Berman!). Amazing combo! Spray the pan and top of the soon-to-be croutons with non-stick cooking spray and bake at 275 until crispy enough for you.

Use tortillas, long thin eggplant or tofu slices as your **pizza base**. Then, instead of cheese, sprinkle a little bit of nutritional yeast over the pizza sauce and veggies. Pizza can be a delivery vehicle for veggies, not cheese! In fact, even if you use regular crust as your pizza base, skip the cheese and add a sprinkling of nutritional yeast. It doesn't actually taste that different from regular pizza.

Whatever you are cooking, ask yourself: Can I **add something green** to that? "Chiffonading" can help. Is that a word? Yes. To "chiffonade" means to stack and roll greens or herbs, like spinach and basil, and slice across the narrow part of the roll. You will have long, thin strips, ideal for pizza, soups, salads and even garnish.

Keep **dehydrated crispy fruit** on hand. Not everyone loves to snack on dehydrated crispy fruit like they do dried fruit. However, it can serve different, but just as convenient, purposes than dried fruit. Rehydrate for an add-in at the last minute when you don't have fresh fruit available or time to deal with it. I throw it in my oatmeal container as I'm running out the door. By the time I get to wherever I am going, it is all soft and yummy, and I have delicious strawberries and bananas in my oatmeal. Dehydrated fruit takes up less room, concentrates the fruit's sweetness and doesn't spoil. It softens quickly in cold cereal and milk. You can also reconstitute it in hot water and use the softened fruit for muffins.

Save time and your eyes. Buy frozen or fresh onions, already **chopped** up for you. It's like having your own sous chef.

Buy **cut up** butternut squash. I know it is expensive. However, when you buy and cut your own, a lot of it seems to go to waste anyway because of the seeds. And then you will actually make and eat it this century. You'll feel so creative now that you don't have to think about all the peeling, chopping and suffering. Roast it, mash it, and put it in soups. Just enjoy not having to cut it!

The KISS [Keep It Simple Stupid] lunch for pre-school kids: beans, veggie and fruit. I have two kids and an OXO set of six small containers. (OXO is a brand found at most home goods stores). I take off the caps and put mandarin oranges (packed in water) in two, canned black beans (that I have rinsed) in another two, and cucumber cut into cute shapes in the last two. I make one sandwich, give one half to each kid, plus 1 container of each of the aforementioned foods, and I have lunch for two little kids. Even after your kids are bigger – and you are bigger – try to keep this system in mind so that you don't get too far from remembering to keep it simple by giving them real food.

Lucky you, I also have a **KISS method for adult lunches** (or dinners on the fly). To quote Dr. Joel Fuhrman, "The salad is the main meal!" A wonderful New York health coach, Marissa Vicario (www.mwahonline.com), taught me the following formula: 4 cups greens, 1 cup grains, 1 cup beans, 1 cup raw or cooked veggies. I always go back to this when I don't know what to eat and when I want to make sure I am eating lean and mean. Greens (cups and cups and you WILL be full!), whole grains (like quinoa or brown rice), legumes (like black beans or chickpeas), and veggies (whatever you've got in the house, whether cooked or raw).

The way to make this fast food is to make sure you have these ingredients at the beginning of the week. Keep a container of a whole grain and a container of beans in the fridge. You can even cut up veggies ahead of time. Make a big batch of healthy and flavorful dressing, too, and for the rest of the week, you have an instant meal whenever you want. If you are trying to lose weight, keep grains to one half cup.

Apple sauce snacks. Squeezees are all the rage right now. They are much more expensive than individual cups, which are in turn much more expensive than a regular ol' jar of apple sauce. Try the little cups as a convenient cost-conscious in between option. For a long time, pre-kids, I only bought apple sauce in the little cups. I did not eat it regularly, and my jar would always get moldy before I could finish it. Also, the little cups are exactly 1/3 of a cup – which is what I would use when substituting apple sauce for oil in a cake mix recipe. Whichever you buy, make sure you are buying apple sauce that only contains apples! Apple juice concentrate and pectin are probably okay. Sugar and artificial sweetener are not. If you do buy a big jar and divvy it into little containers, (we have a frog and a ladybug), the kids will still love it.

If you are cooking for grown-ups or older kids, **one pot meals** are an easy option. Include raw veggies and fruit on the side.

Never again feel like you are "**wasting time**" or like you'd rather be anywhere but the kitchen. If you are about to start a big pile of dishes or need to clean off the counters, and, like me, you are annoyed about it, I have two suggestions.

Start borrowing audio books from the library or subscribe to a service like audible.com. I pay $12.95 per month for a credit for 1 book. I found a mystery thriller series I like and now I enjoy washing the dishes! It is a treat for me to have that time and enjoy a book. It's not like I usually allow myself to sit down and read for pleasure!

Throw something in the oven or on the cooktop. For instance, you can cook potatoes for the week, put rice in the rice cooker or make quinoa on the stove. When you are done cleaning up, you will feel much more accomplished.

Tricks are for Kids!

Turn peanut butter and jelly into "**Elmo heads**" for lunch. I have a cutter that makes Elmo heads and then an Elmo sandwich container. We also have a butterfly sandwich cutter. Depending on your child's favorite animals and characters, you can find anything in the regular grocery store or, of course, online. My mom also uses a big cookie cutter to give my daughter heart shaped sandwiches. (And then the crust is already cut off! An adult can eat that part, so it doesn't go to waste.)

Put out five foods and tell your kids they can **pick any three** they want. You can even make the decision process into a game.

Put some grapes or other healthy food on the kitchen table. Then walk away. **Keep your mouth shut and see what happens.** Kids will usually become curious and eat whatever you have put out. You can even act like you were saving them for something else, but you are being very generous letting them have some anyway.

Bring an apple in the car for yourself. Start eating it. Just wait. Your children will ask you for a bite, and then they will want yours. Then they will both want it and start fighting over the one apple. That's when you "remember" that you happen to have more apples in the car. Just be sure to have one apple for each child or you could have a riot on your hands! This has happened to me!

When you pick up your kids, **bring fresh fruit**, especially cut up watermelon and cantaloupe. They're always hungry and thirsty. If there isn't anything else in the car, they will realize how refreshing and delicious the melon is and gobble up the snack.

Kitchen Equipment

If you think I might as well have two heads for suggesting that any sane person **buy a Vitamix** for hundreds of dollars, any blender will do for a fruit smoothie. Even apples, a fruit you don't usually think of using in a smoothie, will work. However, your green smoothies will not be silky, smooth and fluffy – which I personally find necessary in order to enjoy them. Just sayin'.

I don't ask my kids if they want cucumbers and apples. I ask if they want cucumber and apple SHAPES. **Japanese fruit and vegetable cutters** abound online. Just make sure you understand which size you are buying. Some are appropriate for smaller fruits and veggies and some can only be used with bigger ones. We use a variety of lotus flower blossom shapes although we call some flowers, one a sun, and another a bat. That's what they look like to us!

Not only can you buy a knife that cuts carrots, sweet potatoes and white potatoes into **fun crinkle fries**, you can even buy one that is made for children to use! www.forsmallhands.com

Children will listen to you more when they feel they have power and autonomy, especially around food and the kitchen. The **www.forsmallhands.com** website and catalogue was suggested to us by my children's Montessori school. Children love to use their own whisk, rolling pin and child-safe knives. They will even enjoy sweeping up their crumbs with their child-sized broom and dustpan!

Most of us have seen the expensive "bouquets" of fruit flowers. Did you know you can make your own? I bought a kit for this at the local drug store for $10. It is an activity my daughter and her friends can do forever! Great birthday party activity, too. Instead of decorating cookies with mounds of frosting and sprinkles, they can make their own **fruit flowers** and bouquets – eating cantaloupe, honeydew, watermelon and grapes along the way.

Use that **slow cooker**! If you won't be home for many hours, buy a cheap outlet timer from the drug store or buy an expensive slow cooker with a timing feature. You can even put the ingredients together the night before, put it in the refrigerator, and then take it out and turn it on in the morning. There are many good vegan slow cooker recipe books out there. Also, unlike meat and cheese, vegetables and beans can sit out until the timer turns the slow cooker on – say, five hours before you get home from your 12 hour day. It also makes a lot of food, so you may only need to cook 3 times per week.

Griddle! Never make pancakes and French toast one or two at a time on the cooktop. Use a non-stick plug in griddle and you will save so much time, annoyance and energy. Also, you won't have to scrub a metal pan for two hours or sit there flipping pancakes at the speed of a turtle! More importantly, you won't need to add lots of fat to keep the food from sticking. Just spray a little non-stick spray and you are set.

Buy a cheap **rice cooker**. You don't need anything fancy, but pick one that will also allow you to steam vegetables. I got mine for $20 at a discount home goods store. You can make a quick dinner or pot of rice with so little stress and effort.

Strategies for Clarity

Create a **structure for your meals** (like a fill in the blank book). For example, here is one I have used:
Breakfast: fresh fruit, green smoothie or oatmeal, with nuts or seeds
Lunch: salad with any leftover cooked vegetables, ½ to 1 cup of cooked quinoa, brown rice, or sweet potato, ½ to one cup of beans, homemade salad dressing, 2 cups raw vegetables and 2-4 cups greens.
Dinner: roasted vegetables, sweet potatoes, soup and/or a dish like tofu, brown rice pasta, make your own tacos or cheese-less pizza.

Decide on prep timing, structure, and responsibilities. **Think of cooking like laundry.** Some people prefer a laundry day, where they take care of everything until it is done. Others prefer to throw in a load whenever they have a chance, so that it never feels overwhelming.

Cooking can often be divided into several categories.

- Items that are ready to go, without any or very minimal prep (fruit, nuts, carrots, celery, grape tomatoes).

- Dishes that require time, but not a lot of attention, such as slow roasting a dozen sweet potatoes once or twice a week, making rice or quinoa.

- Dishes that require both time and attention, such as sautéing vegetables on the cook top, gathering and blending ingredients for healthy salad dressing, making a giant green salad to keep ready in the fridge.

Your own tastes, schedule and size and age of your family will influence how you divvy up food duties, among people and over certain days. Healthy food preparation does take time. Once I had kids I understood why people grab dinner at a fast food drive-thru in between school, activities and homework. Thankfully, keeping kosher precludes that from ever being an option for my family.

My solution is to turn food prep time into family time (rather than drudgery or mom alone in the kitchen feeling like she has to do everything) and to make you feel like you already have fast food in your house.

This is accomplished two ways:

- Scheduling food preparation so that you can reach into the fridge and grab healthy options and go.

- Keeping convenient products on hand, like whole fruit, frozen vegetables and ready to eat (canned or frozen) legumes.

Identify the **different meals** your family needs. For instance, if one night a week is filled with activities, you might have to pack everyone's dinner. Some members of the family bring lunch to work and school, while others may need to purchase food and others are home to eat lunch.

As you go through this process, see how you might need to make adjustments. Do you and/or your kids have too many activities? Are there any responsibilities that aren't a top priority right now? Can you delegate anything (family, friends, carpooling or hired help)?

Organizing your food can open many windows of insight into what is or isn't working in your daily life.

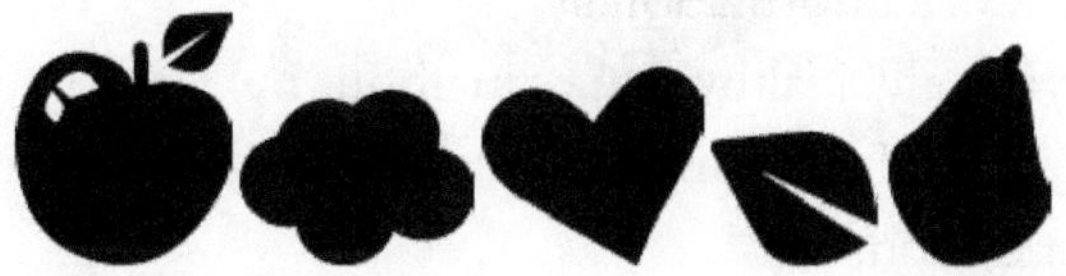

NOW WHAT?

If you are looking for more healthy inspiration, information and recipes, pick *The Healthy Family, Healthy You Cookbook* at www.Amazon.com or www.HealthyFamilyHealthyYou.com.

Want to help your friends and/or community create their own healthy families and a community of support around eating well?

Want to bring valuable information and empowerment to your community, mom's group or your girlfriends?

Looking for personal support and/or help going through the strategies outlined in the book?

You will find more information at www.HealthyFamilyHealthyYou.com about my Girls Night Out events, workshops, fruit funshops for kids, online programs and personal support options.

I hope to connect with you soon!

Yours in health,
Natasha
Natasha@HealthyFamilyHealthyYou.com

END NOTES

[i] Tsukahara N, Ezawa I. [Calcium intake and osteoporosis in many countries]. Clin Calcium. 2001 Feb;11(2):173-7.
[ii] Feskanich D, Willett WC, Colditz GA. Calcium, vitamin D, milk consumption and hip fractures: a prospective study among postmenopausal women. Am J Clin Nutr 2003;77(2): 504-11.
[iii] NOF. "Bone Health Basics." National Osteoporosis Foundation. 2010. http://www.nof.org/aboutosteoporosis/bonebasics/whybonehealth (accessed October 2014).
[iv] Vondracek SF, Hansen LB, McDermott MT. Osteoporosis risk in premenopausal women. Pharmacotherapy. 2009 Mar;29(3):305-17.
Massey LK, Whiting SJ. Caffeine, urinary calcium, calcium metabolism and bone. J. Nutr. 1992 3 Sep;123 (9): 1611-14
Sellmeyer DE, Stone KL, Sebastian A, Cummings SR. A high ratio of dietary animal to vegetable protein increases the rate of bone loss and the risk of fracture in postmenopausal women. Study of Osteoporotic Fracture s Research Group. Am J Clin Nutr. 2001 Jan;73(1):118-22.
Teucher B, Fairweather-Tait S. Dietary sodium as a risk factor for osteoporosis: where is the evidence? Proc Nutr Soc. 2003;62(4):859-866.
Wynn E, Krieg MA, Lanham-New SA, et al. Postgraduate Symposium: Positive influence of nutritional alkalinity on bone health. Proc Nutr Soc. 2010 Feb;69(1):166-73.
[v] Weaver CM, Plawecki KL. Dietary calcium: adequacy of a vegetarian diet. Am J Clin Nutr 1994;59(suppl):1238S-1241S.
[vi] Shea, MK, Booth SL, Update on the role of vitamin K in skeletal health. Nutrition Reviews, 2008. 66(10): p.549-57. Iwamoto J, Sato Y,Takeda T, Matsumoto H. High-dose vitamin K supplementation reduces fracture incidence in postmenopausal women: a review of the lit erature. Nutr Res, 2009. 29(4): p. 221-8.
[vii] University of California - Riverside (2010, July 19). More than half the world's population gets insufficient vitamin D, says biochemist. ScienceDaily. Retrieved October 14, 2014 from http://www.sciencedaily.com¬ /releases/2010/07/100715172042.htm
[viii] Tilyard MW, Spears GF, Thomson J, Dovey S. Treatment of postmenopausal osteoporosis with calcitriol or calcium. N Engl J Med. 1992 Feb 6;326(6):357-62.
[ix] Bischoff-Ferrari, H.A., Optimal serum 25-hydroxyvitamin D levels for multiple health outcomes. Adv Exp Med Biol, 2008. 624: p. 55-71.
[x] ischoff-Ferrari HA, Willett WC. Comment on the IOM Vitamin D and Calcium Recommendations. Harvard School of Public Heal th: The Nutrition Source, 2010.
Zoler ML. High Vitamin D Intake Linked to Reduced Fractures. Family Practice News, 2010(November 16, 2010).
Bischoff-Ferrari HA, Orav EJ, Willett, WC, et al., A Higher Dose of Vitamin D is Required for Hip and Non-vertebral Fracture Prevention: A Pooled Participant-based Meta-analysis of 11 Double-blind RCTs, in The American Society for Bone and Mineral Research 2010 Annual Meeting2010: Toronto, Ontario, Canada.

[xii] Agarwal, U. (2013). Rethinking Red Meat as a Prevention Strategy for Iron Deficiency. *ICAN: Infant, Child, & Adolescent Nutrition.* doi: 10.1177/1941406413491285

[xiii] Campbell, T. C., & Campbell, T. M. (2006). The China study the most comprehensive study of nutrition ever conducted and the startling implications for diet, weight loss and long-term health (p. 103). Dallas, TX: BenBella Books.
[xiv] Campbell, T. C., & Campbell, T. M. (2006). The China study the most comprehensive study of nutrition ever conducted and the startling implications for diet, weight loss and long-term health (p. 7). Dallas, TX: BenBella Books.
[xv] Campbell, T. C., & Campbell, T. M. (2006). The China study the most comprehensive study of nutrition ever conducted and the startling implications for diet, weight loss and long-term health (p. 103). Dallas, TX: BenBella Books.
[xvi] Campbell, T. C., & Campbell, T. M. (2006). The China study the most comprehensive study of nutrition ever conducted and the startling implications for diet, weight loss and long-term health (p. 5). Dallas, TX: BenBella Books.
[xvii] Campbell, T. C., & Campbell, T. M. (2006). The China study the most comprehensive study of nutrition ever conducted and the startling implications for diet, weight loss and long-term health (p. 7). Dallas, TX: BenBella Books.
[xviii] Campbell, T. C., & Campbell, T. M. (2006). The China study the most comprehensive study of nutrition ever conducted and the startling implications for diet, weight loss and long-term health (p. 267). Dallas, TX: BenBella Books.
[xix] Food. (n.d.). Retrieved from http://www.fda.gov/Food/IngredientsPackagingLabeling/LabelingNutrition/ucm073631.htm
[xx] Feloni, R. (2013, November 15). Here's How Many Fast Food Ads American Kids See Each Year. Retrieved from http://www.businessinsider.com/american-children-see-253-mcdonalds-ads-every-year-2013-11
[xxi] Cholesterol Content of Foods. (n.d.). Retrieved from http://www.ucsfhealth.org/education/cholesterol_content_of_foods/
[xxii] Broiler Chicken Industry Key Facts - The National Chicken Council. (n.d.). Retrieved from http://www.nationalchickencouncil.org/about-the-industry/statistics/broiler-chicken-industry-key-facts/.
[xxiii] Tom McDougal. *Poultry Slaughter Procedures.* U.S. Department of Agriculture Food Safety and Inspection Service Office of Field Operations; 1998.
[xxiv] Philpott T. USDA Ruffles Feathers With New Poultry Inspection Policy. *Mother Jones.* April 24, 2013. http://www.motherjones.com/tom-philpott/2013/04/usda-inspectors-poultry-kill-lines-chicken.
[xxv] Tom McDougal. *Poultry Slaughter Procedures.* U.S. Department of Agriculture Food Safety and Inspection Service Office of Field Operations; 1998.
[xxvi] Kindy K. At chicken plants, chemicals blamed for health ailments are poised to proliferate. *The Washington Post.* April 25, 2013. http://articles.washingtonpost.com/2013-04-25/politics/38803667_1_poultry-plants-amanda-hitt-chemicals.
[xxvii] Telesca J. A Closer Look at the FDA Antibiotic Retail Meat Report. *Supermarket News.* March 28, 2013. http://supermarketnews.com/blog/closer-look-fda-antibiotic-retail-meat-report. Accessed May 15, 2013.
[xxviii] Poultry Drug Increases Levels of Toxic Arsenic in Chicken Meat. Johns Hopkins Center for a Livable Future at the Bloomberg School of Public Health. http://www.jhsph.edu/research/centers-and-institutes/johns-hopkins-center-for-a-livable-future/news_events/announcement/2013/toxic_arsenic_chicken_meat.html.

END NOTES

[xxix] Campbell, T. C., & Campbell, T. M. (2006). The China study the most comprehensive study of nutrition ever conducted and the startling implications for diet, weight loss and long-term health (p. 83). Dallas, TX: BenBella Books. (original source) Preston RS, Hayes JR, and Campbell TC. Armstron D, and Doll R. "Environmental factors and cancer incidence and mortality in different countries, with special reference to dietary practices." Int. J. Cancer 15 (1975): 617-631.

[xxx] Barnard, N. (1994). *Foods that cause you to lose weight* (p. 32). McKinney, TX: The Magni Group.

[xxxi] Fuhrman, J. (2014). *The end of dieting: How to live for life* (p. 17). New York, NY: HarperOne.

[xxxii] Barnard, N. (2013, October 10). Chicken Nuggets: Head, Shoulders, Knees, and Toes. Retrieved from http://www.pcrm.org/media/blog/oct2013/chicken-nuggets-head-shoulders-knees-and-toes

[xxxiii] EWG's Guide to BPA. (n.d.). Retrieved October 14, 2014, from http://www.ewg.org/bpa/

[xxxiv] Campbell, T. C., & Campbell, T. M. (2006). The China study the most comprehensive study of nutrition ever conducted and the startling implications for diet, weight loss and long-term health (p. 99). Dallas, TX: BenBella Books.

[xxxv] Campbell, T. C., & Campbell, T. M. (2006). The China study the most comprehensive study of nutrition ever conducted and the startling implications for diet, weight loss and long-term health (p. 101). Dallas, TX: BenBella Books.

[xxxvi] Barnard, N. (1994). *Foods that cause you to lose weight.* McKinney, TX: The Magni Group.

[xxxvii] Ha V, Sievenpiper JL, de Souza RJ, et al. Effect of dietary pulse intake on established therapeutic lipid targets for cardiovascular risk reduction: a systematic review and meta-analysis of randomized controlled trials. *CMAJ.* Published ahead of print April 7, 2014.

[xxxviii] Vergnaud, A., Norat, T., & Romaguera, D., et al. (2010). Meat consumption and prospective weight change in participants of the EPIC-PANACEA study 1,2,3. *Am J Clin Nutr., 92*(2), 398-407. Sabate, J., & Ang, Y. (2009). Nuts and health outcomes: New epidemiologic evidence. *Am J Clin Nutr., 89*(5), 1643S-1648S. Bes-Rastrollo, M., Wedick, N. M., Martinez-Gonzalez, M. A., Li, T. Y., Sampson, L., & Hu, F. B. (2009). Prospective study of nut consumption, long-term weight change, and obesity risk in women. *American Journal of Clinical Nutrition, 89*(6), 1913-1919. doi: 10.3945/ajcn.2008.27276

[xxxix] Fuhrman, J. (2014). *The end of dieting: How to live for life* (p. 118). New York, NY: HarpeRone. His footnote for this is #58 on his page 315. The 0riginal source: Mattes, R. D., & Dreher, M. L. (2010). Nuts and healthy body weight maintenance mechanisms. *Asia Pac J Clin Nutr., 19*, 137-141.

[xli]Healthy at a Glance 2013: OECD Indicators. (2013). Retrieved November 22, 2013, from http://dx.doi.org/10.1787/health_glance-2013-en

Rizzo, N. S., Jaceldo-Siegl, K., Sabate, J., & Fraser, G. E. (2013). Nutrient Profiles of Vegetarian and Nonvegetarian Dietary Patterns. *Journal of the Academy of Nutrition and Dietetics, 113*(12), 1610-1619. doi:10.1016/j.jand.2013.06.349

[xliii] Turner-McGrievy B., Wingard E., Davidson C., Taylor M., Wilcox S. (2013). How Plant based do we need to be to Achieve Weight Loss? Results of the New Dietary Interventions to Enhance the Treatment for Weight Loss (New DIETs) Study [Abstract]. *Obesity Week,* T-53-OR.

[xliv]Kopelman, P. (2000). Obesity as a Medical Problem [Abstract]. *Nature, 404*, 635-643. doi:10.1038/35007508

[xlv] Esposito K., Giugliano F., Di Palo C., et al. (2004). Effect of Lifestyle Changes on Erectile Dysfunction in Obese Men: A Randomized Controlled Trial. *JAMA, 291*(24), 2978-2984. doi:10.1001/jama.291.24.2978.

[xlvi] Mangner N, Scheuermann K, Winzer E, et al. (2014). Childhood Obesity: Impact on Cardiac Geometry and Function. *J Am Coll Cardiol Img, 7*(12), 1198-1205. doi:10.1016/j.jcmg.2014.08.006

[xlvii] Sutherland E. (2008). Obesity and Asthma. *Immunol Allergy Clin North Am*, ***28*(3),** 589-602, ix.. doi: 10.1016/j.iac.2008.03.003

Canoz M., Erdenen F., Uzun H., et al. (2008). The relationship of inflammatory cytokines with asthma and obesity. *Clin Invest Med,* ***31*(6),** E373-379.

Akinbami L., Moorman J., Bailey C., et al. (2012). Trends in Asthma Prevalence, Health Care Use, and Mortality in the United States, 2001-2010. *NCHS Data Brief,* 1-8.

Papoutsakis C., Chondronikola M., Antonogeorgos G., et al. (2014). Associations between Central Obesity and Asthma in Children and Adolescents: A Case Control Study. *J Asthma,* 1-28.

[xlviii] Berentzen N., van Stokkom V., Gehring U., et al. (2014). Associations of Sugar-Containing Beverages with Asthma Prevalence in 11-year-old Children: The PIAMA Birth Cohort. *Eur J Clin Nutr.* doi:10.1038/ejcn.2014.153

Cottrell, L., Neal, W. A., Ice, C., Perez, M. K., & Piedimonte, G. (2011). Metabolic Abnormalities in Children with Asthma. *American Journal of Respiratory and Critical Care Medicine, 183*(4), 441-448. doi:10.1164/rccm.201004-0603OC

Saadeh, D., Salameh, P., Baldi, I., & Raherison, C. (2013). Diet and Allergic Diseases among Population Aged 0 to 18 Years: Myth or Reality? *Nutrients, 5*(9), 3399-3423. doi:10.3390/nu5093399

END NOTES

Jensen, M. E., Gibson, P. G., Collins, C. E., Hilton, J. M., & Wood, L. G. (2013). Diet-induced weight loss in obese children with asthma: A randomized controlled trial. *Clinical & Experimental Allergy, 43*(7), 775-784. doi:10.1111/cea.12115

American Thoracic Society. (2010, May 17). High-fat meals a no-no for asthma patients, researchers find. *ScienceDaily*. Retrieved December 9, 2014 from www.sciencedaily.com/releases/2010/05/100516195534.htm

Go, A. S., Mozaffarian, D., Roger, V. L., & Et al. (2013). Executive Summary: Heart Disease and Stroke Statistics--2013 Update: A Report From the American Heart Association. *Circulation, 127*(1), 143-152. doi:10.1161/CIR.0b013e318282ab8f

[li]Statistics About Diabetes. (2014, June 10). Retrieved December 9, 2014, from http://www.diabetes.org/diabetes-basics/statistics/

Flegal, K. M., Carroll, M. D., Kit, B. K., & Ogden, C. L. (2012). Prevalence of Obesity and Trends in the Distribution of Body Mass Index Among US Adults, 1999-2010. *JAMA: The Journal of the American Medical Association, 307*(5), 491-497. doi:10.1001/jama.2012.39

[liii] Online Library | Articles | Heart Disease is Preventable and Reversible | DrFuhrman.com. (n.d.). Retrieved from http://www.drfuhrman.com/library/heart_disease_preventable_reversible.aspx

Boden, W. E., O'rourke, R. A., & Teo, K. K., & et al. (2007). Optimal Medical Therapy with or without PCI for Stable Coronary Disease. *New England Journal of Medicine, 356*(15), 1503-1516. doi:10.1056/NEJMoa070829

Trikalinos, T. A., Alsheikh-Ali, A. A., Tatsioni, A., & et al. (2009). Percutaneous coronary interventions for non-acute coronary artery disease: A quantitative 20-year synopsis and a network meta-analysis. *The Lancet, 373*(9667), 911-918. doi:10.1016/S0140-6736(09)60319-6

[lv]Hippisley-Cox, J., & Coupland, C. (2010). Unintended effects of statins in men and women in England and Wales: Population based cohort study using the QResearch database. *Bmj, 340*(May19 4), C2197-C2197. doi:10.1136/bmj.c2197

[lvi] Simon S., Black H., Moser M., et al. Cough and ACE Inhibitors. *Arch Intern Med,* ***152,*** 1698-1700.

Bangalore S., Messerli F., Kostis J., et al. (2007**).** Cardiovascular Protection using Beta-Blockers: A Critical Review of the Evidence. *J Am Coll Cardiol,* ***50,*** 563-572.

Gupta, A. K., Dahlof, B., Dobson, J., Sever, P. S., Wedel, H., & Poulter, N. (2008). Determinants of New-Onset Diabetes Among 19,257 Hypertensive Patients Randomized in the Anglo-Scandinavian Cardiac Outcomes Trial-Blood Pressure Lowering Arm and the Relative Influence of Antihypertensive Medication. *Diabetes Care, 31*(5), 982-988. doi:10.2337/dc07-1768

Wassertheil-Smoller, S. (2004). Association Between Cardiovascular Outcomes and Antihypertensive Drug Treatment in Older Women. *JAMA: The Journal of the American Medical Association, 292*(23), 2849-2859. doi:10.1001/jama.292.23.2849

Effects of extended-release metoprolol succinate in patients undergoing non-cardiac surgery (POISE trial): A randomised controlled trial. (2008). *The Lancet, 371*(9627), 1839-1847. doi:10.1016/S0140-6736(08)60601-7

Li, C. I., Daling, J. R., Tang, M. C., Haugen, K. L., Porter, P. L., & Malone, K. E. (2013). Use of Antihypertensive Medications and Breast Cancer Risk Among Women Aged 55 to 74 Years. *JAMA Internal Medicine, 173*(17), 1629. doi:10.1001/jamainternmed.2013.9071

Sipahi, I., Debanne, S. M., Rowland, D. Y., Simon, D. I., & Fang, J. C. (2010). Angiotensin-receptor blockade and risk of cancer: Meta-analysis of randomised controlled trials. *The Lancet Oncology, 11*(7), 627-636. doi:10.1016/S1470-2045(10)70106-6

[lvii]Online Library | Articles | Heart Disease is Preventable and Reversible | DrFuhrman.com. (n.d.). Retrieved from http://www.drfuhrman.com/library/heart_disease_preventable_reversible.aspx

[lviii]Tang W., Wang Z., Fan Y., et al. (2014). Prognostic Value of Elevated Levels of Intestinal Microbe-Generated Metabolite Trimethylamine-N-Oxide in Patients with Heart Failure: Refining the Gut Hypothesis. *J Am Coll Cardiol, 64*, 1908-1914.

[lix]Sugiyama T., Tsugawa Y., Tseng C., Kobayashi Y., Shapiro M. (2014). Different Time Trends of Caloric and Fat Intake between Statin Users and Nonusers among US Adults: Gluttony in the Time of Statins? *JAMA Intern Med., 174*(7), 1038-45. doi: 10.1001/jamainternmed.2014.1927

[lx]Centers for Disease Control. (2010, November). *Colorectal Cancer Statistics.* Retrieved February 2011, from Centers for Disease Control: http://www.cdc.gov/cancer/colorectal/statistics/index.htm

Aune, D., De Stefani, E., Ronco, A., & et al. (2009, November). Legume intake and the risk of cancer: A multisite case-control study in Uruguay. *Cancer Causes Control, 17*(2), 6-12.

Agurs-Collins, T., Smoot, D., Afful, J., & et al. (2006, December). Legume intake and reduced colorectal adenoma risk in African-Americans. *Journal of the National Black Nurses Association, 17*(2), 6-12.

Lanza, E., Hartman, T. J., Albert, P. S., & et al. (2006, July). High dry bean intake and reduced risk of advanced colorectal adenoma recurrence among participants in the polyp prevention trial. *Journal of Nutrition, 136*(7), 1896-1903.
Singh, P. N., & Fraser, G. E. (1998). Dietary risk factors for colon cancer in a low-risk population. *American Journal of Epidemiology*, 148, 761-774.
Faris, M. A., Takruri, H. R., Shomaf, M. S., & Bustani, Y. K. (2009, May). Chemopreventive effect of raw and cooked lentils (Lens culinaris L) and soybeans (Glycine max) against azoxymethane-induced aberrant crypt foci. *Nutrition Research, 29*(5), 355-362.
Williams, E. A., Coxhead, J. M., & Mathers, J. C. (2003, February). Anti-cancer effects of butyrate: use of micro-array technology to investigate mechanisms. *Proceedings of the Nutrition Society, 62*(1), 107-115.
Hamer, H. M., Jonkers, D., Venema, K., & et al. (2008, January 15). The role of butyrate on colonic function. *Alimentary Pharmacology & Therapeutics, 2*, pp. 104-119.
[lxi]*Animal Foods.* (2010). Retrieved from World Cancer Research Fund, American Institute for Cancer Research:
http://www.dietandcancerreport.org/expert_report/recommendations/recommendation_animal_foods.php
[lxii]McCullough, M. L., Gapstur, S. M., Shah, R., Jacobs, E. J., & Campbell, P. T. (2013). Association between red and processed meat intake and mortality among colorectal cancer survivors. *Journal of Clinical Oncology, 31*, 2773-2782.
[lxiii]Link, L. B., Canchola, A. J., Bernstein, L., & et al. (2013, October 9). Dietary patterns and breast cancer risk in the California Teachers Study cohort. *American Journal of Clinical Nutrician*, Epub ahead of print.
[lxiv]Link, L. B., Canchola, A. J., Bernstein, L., & et al. (2013, October 9). Dietary patterns and breast cancer risk in the California Teachers Study cohort. *American Journal of Clinical Nutritian*, Epub ahead of print.
[lxv] Michaud, D. S., Spiegelman, D., & Clinton, S. K. (1999). Fruit and vegetable intake and incidence of bladder cancer in a male prospective cohort. *Journal of the National Cancer Institute, 91*(7), 605-613.
[lxvi]Oranta, O., Pahkala, K., Routtinen, S., & et al. (2013). Infancy-onset dietary counseling of low-saturated-fat diet improves insulin sensitivity in healthy adolescents 15-20 years of age: The Special Turku Coronary Risk Factor Intervention Project (STRIP) study. *Diabetes Care, 36*, 2952-2959.
[lxvii]Diabetologia. (2013, November 11). Higher dietary acid load increases risk of diabetes, study says. *ScienceDaily.* Retrieved November 15, 2014 from
www.sciencedaily.com/releases/2013/11/131111185514.htm
[lxviii]Bao, W., Hu, F. B., Rong, S., & et al. (2013). Predicting risk of Type 2 diabetes mellitus with genetic risk models on the basis of established genome-wide association markers: A systematic review. *American Journal of Epidemiology, 178*, 1197-1207.
[lxix]*Strokes.* (n.d.). Retrieved August 29, 2014 from Dr. Fuhrman:
https://www.drfuhrman.com/disease/Strokes.aspx

[lxx]Lewington, S., Clarke, R., Qizilbash, N., & et al. (2002). Age-specific relevance of usual blood pressure to vascular mortality: A meta-analysis of individual data for one million adults in 61 prospective studies. *Lancet, 360*, 1903-1913.

[lxxi]*Eating to Prevent Alzheimers Disease.* (n.d.). Retrieved November 3, 2014 from Physicians Committee for Responsible Medicine: http://pcrm.org/health/diets/ffl/newsletter/eating-to-prevent-alzheimers-disease

[lxxii]Larsson, S., & Orsini, N. (2014). Red Meat and processed meat consumption and all-cause mortality: a meta-analysis. *American Journal of Epidemiology, 179*(3), 282-9. doi: 10.1093/aje/kwt261

[lxxiii]Lucas, M., Chocano-Bedoya, P., Shulze, M., and et al. (2014). Inflammatory dietary pattern and risk of depression among women. *Brain, Behavior, and Immunity, 36*, 46-53. doi:10.1016/j.bbi.2013.09.014

[lxxiv]Weaver, C. M., & Plawecki, K. L. (1994). Dietary calcium: Adequacy of a vegetarian diet. *American Journal of Clinical Nutrition, 59(suppl)*, 1238S-1241S.

[lxxv]Michaëlsson, K., Wolk, A., Langenskiöld, S., & et al. (2014). Milk intake and risk of mortality and fractures in women and men: Cohort studies. *BMJ, 349, g6015.*

Banks, E., Joshy, G., Abhayaratna, W. P., Kritharies, L., Macdonald, P. S., Korda, R. J., & Chalmers, J. P. (2013). Erectile Dysfunction Severity as a Risk Marker for Cardiovascular Disease Hospitalisation and All-Cause Mortality: A Prospective Cohort Study (S. Ebrahim, Ed.). *PLoS Medicine, 10*(1), E1001372. doi:10.1371/journal.pmed.1001372

Esposito, K. (2004). Effect of Lifestyle Changes on Erectile Dysfunction in Obese Men: A Randomized Controlled Trial. *JAMA: The Journal of the American Medical Association, 291*(24), 2978-2984. doi:10.1001/jama.291.24.2978

[lxxix]Schisterman, E. F., Mumford, S. L., Browne, R. W., Barr, D. B., Chen, Z., & Louis, G. M. (May 20, 2014). *Lipid concentrations and couple fecundity: The LIFE study.* Journal of Clinical Endocrinology and Metabolism. doi: 10.1210/jc.2013-3936

[lxxx]Afeiche, M. (October 14, 2013). *Meat intake and semen parameters among men attending a fertility clinic.* Boston, MA: American Society for Reproductive Medicine.

Afeiche, M., Williams, P. L., & Mediola, J. (2013). Dairy food intake in relation to semen quality and reproductive hormone levels among physically active young men. *Human Reproduction, 28*, 2265-2275.

[lxxxi]Moss, M. (2013). Salt, sugar, fat: How the food giants hooked us. New York: Random House.

[lxxxii]Zhao, J., Moore, A. N., Redell, J. B., & Dash, P. K. (2007). Enhancing Expression of Nrf2-Driven Genes Protects the Blood Brain Barrier after Brain Injury. *Journal of Neuroscience,27*(38), 10240-10248. doi: 10.1523/JNEUROSCI.1683-07.2007

END NOTES

Carter, P., Gray, L. J., Troughton, J., Khunti, K., & Davies, M. J. (2010). Fruit and vegetable intake and incidence of Type 2 diabetes mellitus: Systematic review and meta-analysis. *Bmj,341*(Aug18 4), C4229-C4229. doi: 10.1136/bmj.c4229

Lundberg, J. O., Carlstrom, M., Larsen, F. J., &Weitzberg, E. (2011). Roles of dietary inorganic nitrate in cardiovascular health and disease. *Cardiovascular Research,89*(3), 525-532. doi: 10.1093/cvr/cvq325

[lxxxiii]Higdon, J., Delage, B., Williams, D., & Dashwood, R. (2007). Cruciferous vegetables and human cancer risk: Epidemiologic evidence and mechanistic basis. *Pharmacological Research,55*(3), 224-236. doi:10.1016/j.phrs.2007.01.009

[lxxxiv]Michaud, D. S., Spiegelman, D., Clinton, S. K., Rimm, E. B., Willett, W. C., &Giovannucci, E. L. (1999). Fruit and Vegetable Intake and Incidence of Bladder Cancer in a Male Prospective Cohort. *JNCI Journal of the National Cancer Institute,91*(7), 605-613. doi:10.1093/jnci/91.7.605

[lxxxv]Aune, D., Chan, D. S., Lau, R., Vieira, R., Greenwood, D. C., Kampman, E., &Norat, T. (2011). Dietary fibre, whole grains, and risk of colorectal cancer: Systematic review and dose-response meta-analysis of prospective studies. *Bmj,343*(Nov10 1), D6617-D6617. doi:10.1136/bmj.d6617

[lxxxvi] Jacobs, L. R. (1986). Modification of experimental colon carcinogenesis by dietary fibers. *AdvExp Med Biol, 206*, 105-118.

Gear, J. S., Brodribb, A. J., Ware, A., &Mannt, J. I. (1981). Fibre and bowel transit times. *British Journal of Nutrition,45*(01), 77. doi:10.1079/BJN19810078

[lxxxvii]Atkinson, F. S., Foster-Powell, K., & Brand-Miller, J. C. (2008). International Tables of Glycemic Index and Glycemic Load Values: 2008. *Diabetes Care,31*(12), 2281-2283. doi:10.2337/dc08-1239

[lxxxviii] CWT You Can Do This. (n.d.). Retrieved November 11, 2014, from http%3A%2F%2Fwww.slidesearchengine.com%2Fslide%2F2-cwt-you-can-do-this%20(accessed%2011.11.2014)

[lxxxix]Higginbotham, S., Zhang, Z., Lee, I., Cook, N. R., Giovannucci, E., Buring, J. E., & Liu, S. (2004). Dietary Glycemic Load and Risk of Colorectal Cancer in the Women's Health Study. *JNCI Journal of the National Cancer Institute,96*(3), 229-233. doi:10.1093/jnci/djh020

Michaud, D. S., Fuchs, C. S., & Liu, S. , et al (2005). Dietary glycemic load, carbohydrate, sugar, and colorectal cancer risk in men and women. *Cancer Epidemiol Biomarkers Prev, 14*, 138-147.

Romieu, I., Ferrari, P., Rinaldi, S., & Et al. (2012). Dietary glycemic index and glycemic load and breast cancer risk in the European Prospective Investigation into Cancer and Nutrition (EPIC). *American Journal of Clinical Nutrition,96*(2), 345-355. doi:10.3945/ajcn.111.026724

Dong, J., & Qin, L. (2011). Dietary glycemic index, glycemic load, and risk of breast cancer: Meta-analysis of prospective cohort studies. *Breast Cancer Research and Treatment,126*(2), 287-294. doi:10.1007/s10549-011-1343-3

[xc]Hogervorst, J. G., Schouten, L. J., Konings, E. J., Goldbohm, R. A., & Brandt, P. A. (2007). A Prospective Study of Dietary Acrylamide Intake and the Risk of Endometrial, Ovarian, and Breast Cancer. *Cancer Epidemiology Biomarkers & Prevention,16*(11), 2304-2313. doi:10.1158/1055-9965.EPI-07-0581

Hogervorst, J. G., Schouten, L. J., & Konings, E. J., et al (2008). Dietary acrylamide intake and the risk of renal cell, bladder, and prostate cancer. *Am J ClinNutr, 87*, 1428-1438.

[Expressed In Parts Per Billion (Ppb)]. (n.d.). Center for Science in the Public Interest: Acrylamide Product Charts. *Acrylamide Levels in Dry Cereals.* Retrieved from http://www.cspinet.org/new/pdf/acrylamide_product_charts.pdf

[xci]Gnagnarella, P., Gandini, S., & , La Vecchia, C., et al (2008). Glycemic index, glycemic load, and cancer risk: A meta-analysis. *Am J ClinNutr, 87*, 1793-1801.

[xcii]O'keefe, S. J., Ou, J., Aufreiter, S., & Et al. (2009). Products of the Colonic Microbiota Mediate the Effects of Diet on Colon Cancer Risk. *Journal of Nutrition,139*(11), 2044-2048. doi:10.3945/jn.109.104380

Dronamraju, S. S., Coxhead, J. M., Kelly, S. B., Burn, J., &Mathers, J. C. (2009). Cell kinetics and gene expression changes in colorectal cancer patients given resistant starch: A randomised controlled trial. *Gut,58*(3), 413-420. doi:10.1136/gut.2008.162933

Williams, E. A., Coxhead, J. M., &Mathers, J. C. (2003). Anti-cancer effects of butyrate: Use of micro-array technology to investigate mechanisms. *Proceedings of the Nutrition Society,62*(01), 107-115. doi:10.1079/PNS2002230

Hamer, H. M., Jonkers, D., Venema, K., Vanhoutvin, S., Troost, F. J., &Brummer, R. (2008). Review article: The role of butyrate on colonic function. *Alimentary Pharmacology & Therapeutics,27*(2), 104-119. doi:10.1111/j.1365-2036.2007.03562.x

[xciii]Aune, D., Stefani, E., Ronco, A., Boffetta, P., Deneo-Pellegrini, H., Acosta, G., &Mendilaharsu, M. (2009). Legume intake and the risk of cancer: A multisite case–control study in Uruguay. *Cancer Causes & Control,20*(9), 1605-1615. doi:10.1007/s10552-009-9406-z

Singh, P. N., & Fraser, G. E. (1998). Dietary Risk Factors for Colon Cancer in a Low-risk Population. *American Journal of Epidemiology,148*(8), 761-774. doi:10.1093/oxfordjournals.aje.a009697

[xcivxciv] Schatz, H. S., & Shaiman, S. (2004). If the Buddha came to dinner: How to nourish your body to awaken your spirit. New York: Hyperion.

www.ingramcontent.com/pod-product-compliance
Lightning Source LLC
Chambersburg PA
CBHW050122280326
41933CB00010B/1211
* 9 7 8 0 9 9 6 6 8 4 2 0 0 *